AF350738

Table of Contents

Introduction

# Introduction

## The Power of Healing

Mental health is an integral part of a person's overall well-being, yet it has often been neglected or stigmatized in many communities, particularly within Black households. Understanding mental health's importance and actively seeking therapy when needed can be a transformative experience. Therapy, with its potential for healing and personal growth, offers individuals the tools to navigate emotional, psychological, and social challenges. This is especially critical in Black households, where silence around mental health struggles can often perpetuate cycles of unaddressed trauma and emotional distress.

Therapy provides a structured space for individuals to explore their emotions, experiences, and patterns of behavior, empowering them to gain a deeper understanding of themselves. For Black families, who often endure the compounded stress of societal pressures, economic hardship, and racial discrimination, therapy can offer a release valve, helping to alleviate mental strain. The benefits of therapy can ripple through a family, encouraging open communication, empathy, and support. When normalized, therapy has the power to break the chains of generational trauma and replace them with cycles of healing.

However, despite the potential for healing, therapy remains a taboo subject in many Black households. Societal conditioning and cultural norms often frame vulnerability as weakness, making it difficult for individuals to seek the help they need. Within this context, mental health issues are often ignored or treated with secrecy, leading to long-term emotional suffering. Therapy can transform this landscape by offering a pathway to emotional freedom, one in which mental health becomes a priority and not a source of shame.

The importance of therapy extends beyond individual healing. When one member of a family engages in therapy, the effects can extend outward, improving communication and relationships within the household. Therapy equips individuals with strategies for coping, conflict resolution, and emotional regulation, all of which can have profound effects on family dynamics. In Black households, where systemic challenges often heighten stress and emotional fatigue, these skills are invaluable. As more families engage in therapy, the cultural narrative around mental health can shift, making it more accepted and integrated into daily life.

# Cultural Context and Historical Barriers

## Historical Mistrust of Medical Systems

A significant barrier to therapy in Black communities is the historical mistrust of medical systems. For centuries, Black people have been subjected to mistreatment and exploitation by medical institutions, leaving an indelible mark of distrust. The infamous Tuskegee Syphilis Study, where Black men were deliberately left untreated for syphilis without their knowledge or consent, serves as a glaring example of this betrayal. Additionally, the forced sterilization of Black women and the unethical experiments conducted on enslaved people in the 19th century further deepened the community's mistrust of the medical field.

This distrust was not unwarranted, as these incidents reveal how medical systems have historically marginalized Black individuals, viewing them as subjects for experimentation rather than as patients deserving of care and dignity. The legacy of these abuses still echoes today, creating a reluctance to engage with healthcare services, including mental health therapy. In many Black households, this historical trauma has been passed down, contributing to a deep-seated skepticism of therapy as a form of intervention.

Mistrust of medical institutions extends beyond the historical injustices. Even today, disparities in healthcare access and treatment for Black individuals persist. Studies consistently show that Black patients are less likely to receive adequate mental health care and are often misdiagnosed or under-treated compared to their white counterparts. This systemic bias reinforces the perception that mental health services, including therapy, may not serve Black individuals in a culturally sensitive or equitable manner.

## Generational Trauma and Mental Health

Generational trauma plays a critical role in shaping attitudes toward therapy in Black households. Often referred to as intergenerational trauma, this concept reflects the way in which the emotional and psychological wounds of one generation can be passed down to the next. For Black communities, the trauma of slavery, segregation, and ongoing systemic racism has left a legacy of pain that continues to manifest in the present.

This trauma can appear in various forms, including heightened stress responses, emotional suppression, and a general mistrust of institutions. The pervasive experience of racism in everyday life only adds to this burden, creating a collective wound that is difficult to heal without acknowledging its existence. In many Black households, there is an unspoken understanding of this trauma, but it is rarely addressed directly. Instead, the pain is often internalized or expressed through behaviors such as anger, withdrawal, or substance abuse.

The reluctance to confront these deep-seated traumas is partly due to cultural norms that prioritize strength and resilience. The "strong Black man" and "strong Black woman" tropes encourage individuals to bear their emotional burdens in silence, reinforcing the idea that seeking help is a sign of weakness. While resilience is indeed a valued quality, it can become detrimental when it discourages people from addressing their mental health needs.

Therapy can play a pivotal role in breaking the cycle of generational trauma by providing a space to explore these inherited wounds. For Black households, therapy offers an opportunity to confront and process the emotional scars that have been passed down through generations. By acknowledging and addressing this trauma, individuals can begin to heal, paving the way for healthier relationships and emotional well-being for future generations.

**Systemic Racism and Socioeconomic Barriers**
Systemic racism is another critical factor that shapes the relationship between Black households and therapy. Structural inequalities,

such as inadequate access to quality healthcare, education, and employment opportunities, create a range of stressors that disproportionately affect Black communities. These stressors, combined with the ongoing experience of racial discrimination, contribute to the development of mental health issues such as depression, anxiety, and post-traumatic stress disorder (PTSD).

Unfortunately, the same systems that create these stressors often fail to provide adequate support for mental health. Black individuals are less likely to have access to mental health services, either due to financial constraints or a lack of culturally competent providers. The cost of therapy, compounded by economic disparities, can make it inaccessible for many Black families, particularly those in low-income communities.

Even when therapy is accessible, Black individuals may encounter therapists who are not adequately trained in cultural competence. This can lead to misunderstandings, misdiagnoses, or a lack of trust between the therapist and the client. A therapist who does not fully understand the cultural and societal context in which their Black clients live may struggle to provide effective support, further reinforcing the notion that therapy is not a viable option for Black individuals.

Culturally competent therapy is crucial for addressing the unique mental health needs of Black individuals and families. This form of therapy acknowledges the cultural, social, and historical factors that influence mental health in Black communities. It also involves creating a therapeutic space that is free from judgment and stigma, where individuals can openly discuss their experiences with racism, cultural identity, and generational trauma.

## Stigmatization of Therapy in Black Households

The stigma surrounding therapy in Black households is one of the most significant barriers to its acceptance. For many, therapy is seen as a sign of failure or weakness, particularly in a cultural context where strength and resilience are highly valued. Admitting to mental health struggles is often equated with being unable to "handle life," and seeking help is sometimes viewed as betraying the family or community's expectations of perseverance.

Additionally, mental health challenges are frequently minimized or dismissed within Black families. Expressions like "You'll be fine," "Pray about it," or "Just toughen up" are commonly used to brush aside signs of emotional distress. These phrases, though often well-meaning, contribute to a culture of silence around mental health issues. When therapy is dismissed as unnecessary or ineffective, individuals are left to cope with their struggles alone, which can lead to more severe mental health problems over time.

This stigmatization of therapy is also tied to broader societal expectations. Black individuals are often expected to perform emotional labor both within their communities and in the wider world, particularly in contexts where they are navigating predominantly white spaces. The pressure to appear unflappable, even in the face of racism and discrimination, can make it difficult to acknowledge and address emotional vulnerabilities. Therapy challenges these expectations by encouraging individuals to confront their pain, but this can feel risky in a world that often demands emotional stoicism from Black people.

**Shifting the Cultural Narrative**

To make therapy more accepted and normalized in Black households, it is essential to shift the cultural narrative around mental health. This begins with education and awareness, helping individuals understand that mental health is just as important as physical health and that seeking therapy is a proactive step toward healing. By reframing therapy as an act of strength, rather than weakness, Black families can begin to break the cycle of silence and stigmatization.

Public figures and influencers who openly discuss their experiences with therapy can play a powerful role in shifting this narrative. When celebrities, athletes, and other prominent Black individuals speak candidly about their mental health journeys, they help to normalize therapy within the community. Their stories can inspire others to seek help, showing that vulnerability is not a sign of failure but a pathway to healing.

Additionally, integrating conversations about mental health into everyday life can help reduce the stigma surrounding therapy. Schools, churches, and community organizations can play a vital role in promoting mental health education and providing resources for those in need. By creating spaces where mental health is openly discussed and supported, these institutions can help Black families feel more comfortable seeking therapy.

## Conclusion

The power of healing through therapy cannot be overstated, particularly in Black households where mental health issues are often met with silence or stigma. Therapy offers a transformative opportunity to address the historical, cultural, and systemic barriers that have prevented Black individuals and families from seeking the care they need. By acknowledging the importance of mental health, confronting generational trauma, and shifting the cultural narrative, Black families can begin to embrace therapy as a valuable tool for healing and growth.

Breaking the silence around mental health in Black households is not only necessary for individual well-being but also for the collective healing of the community. Therapy provides a space for Black individuals to confront their pain, process their experiences, and develop the tools to navigate life's challenges with resilience and self-compassion. As the conversation around mental health evolves, the hope is that therapy will become not only more accepted but also celebrated as an essential part of the journey toward emotional freedom and empowerment.

# Chapter 1: Understanding the Cultural Stigma

## Why Therapy is Still Taboo in Many Black Homes

Mental health care, particularly therapy, has long been a topic surrounded by stigma and resistance in many Black households. To fully understand why therapy remains taboo, it is necessary to explore the complex intersection of cultural beliefs, strong religious faith, and the societal expectations surrounding Black strength. These factors create a unique context where seeking help for mental health challenges is often seen as unnecessary or even shameful. By examining these cultural barriers, we can gain insight into why therapy has not yet been fully embraced and explore the steps necessary to break this cycle of resistance.

# Cultural Beliefs Surrounding Mental Health

For generations, many Black families have been conditioned to view emotional vulnerability and mental health struggles as a sign of personal weakness or failure. This belief is deeply ingrained in cultural norms that prioritize strength, resilience, and the ability to endure hardship. Black people, particularly in the United States, have a long history of surviving adversity, from slavery and segregation to ongoing systemic racism and economic inequality. In this context, "keeping it together" and appearing unbreakable are seen as crucial survival strategies.

This cultural emphasis on strength often discourages individuals from admitting that they need help, let alone seeking therapy. Asking for assistance, especially when it comes to emotional or psychological challenges, is frequently viewed as a failure to live up to the standards set by one's ancestors and community. This pressure to "handle everything" without external support can prevent individuals from acknowledging mental health issues and can lead to the suppression of emotions.

The stigma around therapy in Black households is also reinforced by misconceptions about what therapy entails. Many people within the community still view therapy as something exclusively for individuals who are "crazy" or deeply troubled, rather than as a tool for emotional well-being and personal growth. Therapy is often misunderstood as a last resort, only to be considered in extreme circumstances, rather than as a proactive way to address everyday stressors, anxiety, or emotional challenges. This misunderstanding leads to further reluctance to explore therapy as a viable option for mental health care.

## The Role of Strong Religious Faith

Religion has historically played a central role in Black culture, providing a source of strength, resilience, and community in the face of adversity. For many Black families, the church is not just a place of worship but a cultural and social hub, where individuals find comfort, connection, and support. Black religious traditions have long emphasized faith, prayer, and reliance on God as essential components of coping with life's challenges. While this deep faith has provided solace for countless individuals, it has also, at times, contributed to the stigmatization of therapy and other mental health services.

In many Black households, the response to mental health struggles is often, "Pray about it." This phrase encapsulates the belief that turning to God and relying on spiritual guidance will provide the necessary healing and support. While faith can undoubtedly be a powerful source of emotional resilience, it can also create a barrier to seeking therapy when individuals believe that prayer alone should be enough to resolve their mental health challenges.

This reliance on prayer is sometimes accompanied by a mistrust of mental health professionals, who may be viewed as outsiders to the faith or as promoting solutions that are not spiritually aligned. Some individuals within Black religious communities may even believe that seeking therapy is a sign of weak faith or a lack of trust in God's ability to heal. This belief can lead to feelings of guilt or shame for individuals who consider seeking therapy, as it may be interpreted as doubting the power of their religion.

However, it's important to note that faith and therapy do not have to be mutually exclusive. In fact, many therapists recognize the importance of integrating a client's religious beliefs into their treatment plans. By acknowledging the role of spirituality in mental health, therapists can help individuals see therapy as a complement to their faith, rather than a contradiction of it. Unfortunately, the perception that therapy and religion are incompatible continues to persist in many Black households, reinforcing the cultural stigma surrounding mental health care.

## The "Strong Black Person" Trope

One of the most pervasive cultural factors contributing to the resistance to therapy in Black communities is the "strong Black person" trope. This social construct idealizes Black individuals as resilient, unbreakable, and capable of enduring immense hardship without showing vulnerability. The origins of this trope can be traced back to slavery and the dehumanizing conditions that Black people were forced to endure. Under these conditions, survival often depended on suppressing emotions, enduring pain in silence, and presenting a façade of strength in the face of unimaginable suffering.

This image of strength has been passed down through generations and has become an integral part of Black identity. While resilience is an admirable and necessary trait, the "strong Black person" trope can be harmful when it discourages individuals from acknowledging their emotional needs. Many Black people feel pressure to live up to this ideal, believing that admitting to mental health struggles would be seen as a betrayal of their cultural legacy.

For Black women, this pressure is often compounded by the "strong Black woman" archetype, which portrays Black women as caretakers who must constantly sacrifice their own well-being for the sake of others. This stereotype reinforces the expectation that Black women should be able to manage both their own challenges and the challenges of their families without complaint. The "superwoman" role, while culturally celebrated, can lead to emotional burnout and prevent Black women from seeking therapy when they are struggling.

Similarly, Black men face their own version of the strength trope, which is tied to traditional notions of masculinity. In many Black households, men are expected to be the providers and protectors, roles that often discourage emotional expression. The cultural expectation of stoicism and emotional control can make it particularly difficult for Black men to acknowledge their mental health needs. Vulnerability is often equated with weakness, and many Black men internalize the belief that therapy is not a valid option for them.

The pressure to maintain the appearance of strength can also manifest in the ways Black individuals respond to stress and trauma. Rather than seeking therapy, many people turn to other coping mechanisms, such as substance abuse, overworking, or emotional suppression. These behaviors, while often seen as a way of "keeping it together," can have long-term negative effects on mental health and well-being. By continuing to equate strength with emotional suppression, the "strong Black person" trope perpetuates the cultural stigma against therapy and prevents many individuals from seeking the help they need.

# The Role of Family Structure and Generational Trauma

## Family Structure in Black Households

The structure of Black families often plays a crucial role in shaping attitudes toward mental health and therapy. Family dynamics in Black households are frequently influenced by cultural values such as collectivism, loyalty, and interdependence. These values can be a source of strength and resilience but can also contribute to the reluctance to seek therapy, as mental health struggles are often viewed as a private family matter that should be handled within the household.

In many Black families, the extended family is a central part of daily life. Grandparents, aunts, uncles, cousins, and other relatives often play significant roles in raising children and providing emotional support. This extended family structure can create a sense of community and shared responsibility, but it can also make it difficult for individuals to seek help outside of the family unit. There may be a belief that airing personal struggles to a therapist or outsider is a betrayal of the family's loyalty and trust.

Additionally, within Black families, the roles of mothers and fathers are often shaped by cultural expectations that reinforce the "strong Black person" trope. Mothers, particularly in single-parent households, are often expected to be the emotional backbone of the family, juggling work, childcare, and emotional support for their children without showing signs of struggle. Fathers, meanwhile, are expected to provide financial stability and emotional strength, even in the face of their own challenges. These gendered expectations can discourage both parents from seeking therapy, as doing so may be seen as failing to fulfill their roles.

## Generational Trauma: Passing Down the Pain

Generational trauma, also known as intergenerational trauma, refers to the ways in which the psychological effects of trauma experienced by one generation can be passed down to the next. In Black communities, the legacy of slavery, segregation, and systemic racism has left deep emotional wounds that continue to affect individuals and families today. This trauma is not limited to the direct experiences of discrimination and violence; it also includes the psychological toll of living in a society that consistently devalues Black lives.

The trauma experienced by ancestors can manifest in later generations through behaviors, attitudes, and emotional responses that are shaped by this historical context. For example, the fear and anxiety that many Black parents feel for their children's safety in a racially biased society can be traced back to the trauma of slavery and segregation, where the lives of Black children were often in danger. This generational fear can lead to heightened stress and anxiety in

Black families, which may go unaddressed due to the cultural stigma around therapy.

Generational trauma can also contribute to the way mental health is perceived within Black households. Many Black families have learned to cope with trauma by normalizing suffering and emotional suppression. This normalization of pain, passed down through generations, can make it difficult for individuals to recognize when they are struggling with their mental health. Instead of seeking therapy, individuals may internalize the belief that emotional suffering is simply a part of life that must be endured.

The effects of generational trauma are further compounded by ongoing experiences of systemic racism, which continues to create stress, anxiety, and emotional pain for Black individuals. Microaggressions, racial profiling, and economic inequality are just a few of the ways that racism manifests in everyday life, contributing to mental health challenges that are often left unaddressed. The weight of generational trauma, combined with the daily stressors of racism, creates a unique mental health burden that therapy could help alleviate—if it were not for the cultural stigma that prevents many Black individuals from seeking help.

## Breaking the Cycle: The Path Forward

To address the cultural stigma surrounding therapy in Black households, it is essential to break the cycle of generational trauma and challenge the societal expectations that equate strength with emotional suppression. This begins with acknowledging the deep-seated cultural beliefs that have contributed to the resistance to therapy and recognizing that seeking help is not a sign of weakness but a courageous step toward healing.

Black families must be empowered to redefine what it means to be strong. True strength lies not in the ability to endure pain in silence but in the willingness to seek help when it is needed. By challenging the "strong Black person" trope and encouraging emotional vulnerability, individuals can begin to break down the barriers that have prevented previous generations from accessing mental health care.

At the same time, it is important to honor the role of faith and spirituality in Black culture. Rather than viewing therapy as incompatible with religion, it is possible to integrate both practices into a holistic approach to mental health. Therapists who work with Black clients should be aware of the importance of spirituality and be open to incorporating a client's religious beliefs into their treatment plans.

Finally, addressing generational trauma requires a concerted effort to provide mental health education and resources to Black communities. By increasing access to culturally competent therapists and providing opportunities for open dialogue about mental health, Black families can begin to heal from the traumas of the past and create a new legacy of emotional well-being for future generations.

# Chapter 2: The Intersection of Faith and Therapy

## Blending Faith with Mental Health Practices

For many Black families, faith serves as a cornerstone of life. The church has historically provided more than just spiritual guidance; it has been a place of solace, community, and resistance to systemic oppression. Faith and religion have empowered Black people to persevere through centuries of adversity, from slavery to segregation to modern-day racism. In Black households, religious faith is often viewed as the ultimate source of healing, emotional strength, and problem-solving. However, when it comes to mental health, the question arises: How can faith coexist with therapeutic practices? Are the two at odds, or can they be integrated to support comprehensive emotional and mental well-being?

The intersection of faith and therapy is particularly significant in Black communities, where mental health challenges are often met with religious solutions. Statements like "pray about it" or "give it to God" reflect the deep belief that spiritual healing can resolve even the most complex emotional issues. While prayer and religious practices can certainly offer comfort and a sense of peace, mental health care requires more than just faith—it often requires professional intervention. Blending faith with therapy, rather than seeing them as separate or competing paths, can offer a holistic approach to mental health in Black households.

## The Role of Religion in Black Communities

To understand the intersection of faith and therapy, it is important to first acknowledge the significant role that religion plays in Black communities. Historically, the Black church has been much more than just a religious institution—it has functioned as a center of social and political activism, a refuge from racial oppression, and a source of communal strength. For many Black people, their religious identity is intertwined with their cultural identity. The church has offered a safe space where the congregation can gather to pray, seek counsel, and support each other in times of hardship.

Because of the centrality of religion, it is not uncommon for mental health struggles to be addressed first and foremost through faith. This response is understandable when considering the many benefits that spiritual practices can offer. Prayer, meditation, and community worship can help reduce anxiety, increase feelings of hope, and promote emotional resilience. For many, their faith is the first place they turn to when faced with emotional challenges, and this reliance on faith can offer genuine psychological benefits.

However, when religious practices are seen as the only solution to mental health struggles, it can prevent individuals from seeking additional help from professionals. There is a prevailing belief in some Black households that if one has enough faith, God will provide healing for all aspects of life, including mental health. This mindset can lead to feelings of guilt or shame when individuals find that prayer alone is not enough to alleviate their emotional struggles. The pressure to maintain a strong faith, combined with the cultural stigma surrounding therapy, can prevent people from exploring other avenues of healing, such as counseling or psychiatric care.

## The Misconception That Faith and Therapy Are Incompatible

One of the primary barriers to blending faith with therapy is the misconception that the two are mutually exclusive. This belief is rooted in the idea that seeking help outside of one's religious community, particularly from a secular therapist, is somehow a sign of weak faith or an act of disloyalty to God. In some religious circles, mental health issues are seen not as psychological or emotional challenges but as spiritual battles. Depression, anxiety, and other mental health conditions may be interpreted as a lack of faith or even as evidence of spiritual attacks. As a result, individuals are often encouraged to strengthen their relationship with God, pray more fervently, or engage in spiritual rituals rather than seek professional mental health care.

This misconception overlooks the fact that therapy and faith are not inherently at odds. In fact, many therapists, particularly those who work with religious clients, are trained to incorporate a person's spiritual beliefs into their treatment plans. Therapy does not require an abandonment of faith; rather, it can be used to complement religious practices. Mental health professionals who respect and understand their clients' religious beliefs can help create a space where both faith and therapy are valued as important tools for healing.

It is also important to note that not all forms of therapy are secular in nature. Some therapists specialize in faith-based counseling, which integrates spiritual teachings and mental health practices. This type of therapy can be especially appealing to individuals who want to seek help but feel that secular therapy may not align with their religious values. By offering a space where faith is central to the therapeutic process, faith-based therapy provides an opportunity for individuals to address their mental health challenges without feeling that they are compromising their religious identity.

## How Mental Health Professionals Can Incorporate Spirituality into Therapy

For therapists who work with Black clients from religious backgrounds, it is essential to recognize the importance of faith in their lives. Rather than dismissing or downplaying the role of religion, mental health professionals should strive to incorporate a client's spiritual beliefs into their therapeutic approach. This can be done in several ways:

1. **Active Listening and Respect for Religious Beliefs:** One of the most important steps a therapist can take is to listen carefully to a client's beliefs about faith and healing. Therapists should not assume that a client's religious beliefs are an obstacle to therapy but should instead view them as an important aspect of the client's identity and worldview. By showing respect for a client's faith, therapists can create an atmosphere of trust and openness, where clients feel comfortable

discussing both their spiritual and emotional struggles.

2.  **Exploring the Intersection of Faith and Mental Health:** Therapists can help clients explore how their faith can be a source of strength and resilience in their mental health journey. For many religious individuals, their faith provides them with a sense of purpose, hope, and meaning, all of which can be valuable in overcoming mental health challenges. Therapists can work with clients to identify how their spiritual practices—such as prayer, meditation, or attending religious services—can be integrated into their coping strategies.

3.  **Addressing Religious Guilt or Shame:** Some clients may feel guilt or shame for seeking therapy, especially if they have been taught that prayer should be sufficient for healing. Therapists can help clients navigate these feelings by offering a compassionate and non-judgmental space to explore the relationship between their faith and their mental health needs. By reframing therapy as a form of self-care that is not in conflict with faith, therapists can help clients understand that seeking help is not a sign of weak faith but a step toward holistic healing.

4.  **Collaborating with Religious Leaders:** In some cases, it may be helpful for therapists to collaborate with a client's religious leaders, particularly if the client values their

guidance and sees them as an important part of their support system. By working together, therapists and religious leaders can provide a more comprehensive approach to mental health care that honors both the client's spiritual and psychological needs. This collaboration can also help reduce the stigma around therapy within religious communities, as religious leaders can serve as advocates for mental health care.

5. **Using Spiritual Language and Metaphors:** Therapists can also incorporate spiritual language and metaphors into their therapeutic approach to better align with a client's religious framework. For example, when discussing coping mechanisms or strategies for healing, therapists might use terms like "faith journey," "spiritual growth," or "God's plan" to make the therapy process feel more relevant and accessible to religious clients. By speaking in terms that resonate with a client's faith, therapists can bridge the gap between spirituality and mental health care.

# Creating Space for Both Prayer and Professional Help

For Black families, the challenge often lies in finding a balance between relying on spiritual practices, such as prayer, and seeking professional help for mental health challenges. Rather than viewing therapy and faith as competing solutions, it is possible to create space for both. The key is understanding that prayer and therapy can serve different but complementary roles in the healing process.

Prayer is a deeply personal and spiritual practice that can provide comfort, clarity, and a sense of connection to a higher power. For many individuals, prayer is a way to process emotions, seek guidance, and find peace in the midst of life's challenges. However, while prayer can be a powerful tool for emotional well-being, it is not a substitute for professional mental health care. Therapy, on the other hand, offers a structured approach to addressing mental health issues, providing individuals with the tools and strategies needed to cope with emotional challenges, trauma, and stress.

## Examples of Individuals Who Combine Faith and Mental Health Treatment

There are many examples of individuals who have successfully blended faith and therapy to create a holistic approach to mental health care. These stories serve as powerful reminders that faith and therapy can coexist and that seeking professional help does not diminish one's spiritual beliefs.

1. **Sarah's Story: Faith-Based Counseling for Depression** Sarah, a devout Christian, struggled with depression for several years but resisted seeking therapy because she believed that her faith should be enough to sustain her. She attended church regularly, prayed daily, and sought guidance from her pastor, but her depression persisted. Eventually, Sarah decided to try faith-based counseling, where her therapist integrated biblical teachings into the therapeutic process. Through this approach, Sarah was able to address her depression while strengthening her relationship with God. She found that therapy helped her develop coping strategies that complemented her spiritual practices, allowing her to manage her depression while maintaining her faith.

2. **James's Story: Healing from Trauma with Therapy and Prayer** James, a Black man in his mid-30s, experienced trauma in his childhood that left him emotionally scarred. He was raised in a deeply religious household where therapy was viewed as unnecessary because "God could heal all wounds." Despite his faith, James found himself struggling with anxiety and panic attacks as an adult. Eventually, he decided to seek therapy, but he made it clear to his therapist that his faith was an essential part of his healing process. His therapist respected his religious beliefs and encouraged him to continue praying while

also working through his trauma in therapy. By combining prayer with therapeutic techniques like cognitive-behavioral therapy (CBT),James was able to process his trauma and find peace.

3. **Aisha's Story: Balancing Spirituality and Mental Health** Aisha, a mother of three, was overwhelmed with stress and anxiety as she tried to balance her work, family, and community responsibilities. She often turned to prayer for comfort but found that it was not enough to alleviate her anxiety. After a particularly challenging year, Aisha decided to seek therapy while continuing her spiritual practices. Her therapist encouraged her to use prayer as a tool for mindfulness, helping her to ground herself before and after therapy sessions. Aisha found that by creating space for both prayer and therapy, she could address her anxiety while nurturing her spiritual growth. She began to view therapy as a means of self-care, understanding that caring for her mental health was essential to being a strong and present mother.

## Conclusion

The intersection of faith and therapy presents a unique opportunity for Black families to engage in a holistic approach to mental health. By blending spiritual practices with professional support, individuals can navigate their emotional struggles while honoring their religious beliefs. Mental health professionals play a vital role in this process by respecting and incorporating a client's faith into therapy.

As more Black families begin to recognize the value of seeking professional help while maintaining their spiritual practices, the stigma surrounding therapy can be reduced. The journey to healing is not a solitary one; it is a multifaceted process that includes prayer, community, and professional guidance. By creating space for both faith and therapy, Black households can foster a culture of emotional well-being that honors their past while paving the way for a healthier future.

# Chapter 3: Rewriting the Narrative

## Redefining Strength in Vulnerability

In many Black communities, the cultural norm of equating strength with emotional suppression has shaped generations of attitudes toward mental health. The notion that being strong means never showing vulnerability or admitting to emotional struggles is deeply embedded in the collective consciousness. For centuries, Black individuals, particularly in the United States, have had to navigate an environment filled with systemic racism, social oppression, and discrimination. In response to this ongoing adversity, resilience has been celebrated as a vital survival tool, and this resilience has often been synonymous with silence. But this narrative, while well-intentioned, has its costs. As we move forward, it's critical to redefine strength in a way that embraces vulnerability as an essential part of emotional and mental health.

# The Cultural Narrative of Strength

The cultural narrative of strength in Black households is often intertwined with survival. Historically, Black families endured slavery, segregation, and structural racism, and being able to withstand unimaginable emotional and physical pain became a badge of honor. The pressure to be strong, whether for oneself or for one's family, became a cultural expectation passed down through generations. As a result, showing vulnerability—especially when it comes to mental health—has often been seen as a weakness or as failing to live up to the historical strength of ancestors.

This cultural expectation has been particularly heavy for Black men and women. For Black men, the image of strength is often tied to traditional notions of masculinity, where emotional expression is viewed as a threat to one's manhood. For Black women, the "strong Black woman" trope has imposed the expectation that they must endure the emotional labor of both themselves and their families without complaint. This pressure to constantly "keep it together" is exhausting and often leads to emotional burnout.

But it's important to recognize that this narrative of strength through silence is not sustainable. Suppressing emotions does not make them disappear; rather, it amplifies them over time, leading to stress, anxiety, depression, and other mental health challenges. This cycle of emotional suppression, passed down from one generation to the next, can have long-lasting impacts on family dynamics, relationships, and personal well-being. As we rewrite the narrative, we must begin to redefine what it means to be strong by embracing vulnerability as an act of courage.

## The Power of Vulnerability

Vulnerability is not the opposite of strength—it is a deeper form of strength. It takes courage to acknowledge one's emotions, to sit with discomfort, and to admit when help is needed. Asking for help, whether from a therapist, a trusted friend, or a family member, requires a level of self-awareness and humility that is deeply powerful. Vulnerability is not about being weak; it is about being authentic and honest with oneself.

In redefining strength, we must challenge the idea that vulnerability is something to be feared or avoided. In fact, vulnerability allows individuals to connect more deeply with themselves and with others. It opens the door to healing by creating a space for emotional expression, reflection, and growth. When Black individuals allow themselves to be vulnerable, they are not betraying the legacy of strength that has been passed down to them; they are expanding on it, creating a new model of resilience that includes emotional health as a priority.

This shift in narrative is particularly important in Black households, where silence around mental health can prevent healing and create a culture of emotional isolation. By modeling vulnerability, parents and caregivers can teach younger generations that asking for help is not something to be ashamed of but something to be proud of. Vulnerability fosters emotional intelligence, empathy, and open communication, which are all essential components of mental well-being.

## Courage in Seeking Help

Asking for help is one of the bravest acts a person can take. It requires breaking through the cultural conditioning that tells us we must manage everything on our own. For many Black individuals, the decision to seek therapy is not just about addressing a personal mental health issue; it is also about challenging deeply ingrained cultural norms. The act of seeking help, therefore, becomes an act of resistance— resisting the idea that strength means silence, and instead embracing the idea that strength comes from self-care and emotional well-being.

Therapy, in this context, is not just a tool for personal healing but a revolutionary act that challenges the harmful norms that have kept Black individuals from seeking the support they deserve. It is a declaration that mental health is just as important as physical health and that taking care of one's emotional and psychological well-being is a vital part of thriving.

In rewriting the narrative, we must celebrate those who have had the courage to seek help. Whether it is through therapy, support groups, or community-based mental health programs, those who embrace their vulnerability and ask for help are laying the groundwork for a new cultural understanding of strength.

# Breaking Myths: "Therapy is for the Weak"

One of the most pervasive myths that persist in Black households is the belief that therapy is only for the weak or for people who are "crazy." This misconception has been a significant barrier to mental health treatment, preventing countless individuals from seeking the help they need. However, as we rewrite the narrative around mental health, it is essential to dispel these myths and replace them with a more accurate understanding of therapy and its benefits.

## Myth 1: Therapy is Only for People with Severe Mental Illness

One of the most common myths about therapy is that it is only for people who have severe mental health conditions, such as schizophrenia or bipolar disorder. While therapy is certainly beneficial for individuals with these conditions, it is by no means limited to them. In fact, therapy is a powerful tool for anyone dealing with a wide range of life challenges, including stress, anxiety, depression, grief, relationship issues, and personal growth. It is not necessary to wait until a crisis occurs to seek therapy; in many cases, early intervention can prevent more serious mental health issues from developing.

For many Black individuals, the belief that therapy is only for people with severe mental illness can create a barrier to accessing care. They may feel that their struggles are not "serious enough" to warrant professional help or that they should be able to handle their challenges on their own. This mindset can lead to prolonged suffering and untreated mental health issues.

Therapy should be viewed as a proactive form of self-care, not just as a last resort. Whether someone is dealing with everyday stressors or more significant life transitions, therapy provides a space for individuals to explore their emotions, gain insight into their behaviors, and develop strategies for coping. By normalizing therapy as a tool for emotional well-being, we can break down the myth that it is only for people with severe mental health conditions.

## Myth 2: Therapy is a Sign of Weakness

Another prevalent myth is the idea that seeking therapy is a sign of weakness. This belief is particularly harmful because it reinforces the cultural expectation that strength means handling everything on one's own. In Black communities, where resilience is highly valued, this myth can prevent individuals from acknowledging their mental health needs and seeking the support they deserve.

The reality is that therapy is not about weakness —it is about self-awareness, growth, and healing. It takes courage to admit when something is not working and to seek help in addressing it. Therapy provides individuals with the tools to better understand themselves, to process their emotions, and to develop healthier coping mechanisms. Far from being a sign of weakness, therapy is an act of strength and self-care.

One way to challenge this myth is by highlighting stories of individuals who have used therapy as a way to strengthen their emotional resilience. Public figures like Taraji P. Henson, Charlamagne Tha God, and Gabrielle Union have openly discussed their experiences with therapy, helping to destigmatize mental health treatment in Black communities. By sharing these stories, we can show that therapy is not a sign of failure but a path to empowerment.

## Myth 3: Therapy Doesn't Work for Black People

There is also a persistent belief in some Black communities that therapy doesn't "work" for Black people, either because therapists don't understand the cultural context or because the therapeutic process itself is seen as incompatible with the Black experience. This myth is rooted in historical mistrust of medical institutions, as well as a lack of representation in the mental health field. Many Black individuals have encountered therapists who are not culturally competent and who fail to understand the unique challenges that come with being Black in America. As a result, they may leave therapy feeling misunderstood or invalidated.

While it is true that cultural competence is essential for effective therapy, this does not mean that therapy as a whole is ineffective for Black individuals. There are many Black therapists and culturally competent therapists who are trained to understand the specific needs of Black clients. Moreover, therapy can be tailored to meet the individual needs of each client, incorporating cultural, religious, and social factors into the treatment plan.

In recent years, there has been a growing movement to increase access to culturally competent mental health care for Black communities. Initiatives like the Therapy for Black Girls directory and the National Queer and Trans Therapists of Color Network are helping to connect individuals with therapists who understand their cultural background and can provide the support they need. By increasing access to culturally competent care, we can break down the myth that therapy is ineffective for

Black people and encourage more individuals to seek help.

## Myth 4: Therapy is Too Expensive and Inaccessible

Cost is often cited as a major barrier to therapy, particularly for individuals in low-income communities. The belief that therapy is too expensive and inaccessible can prevent many Black individuals from even considering it as an option. While it is true that therapy can be costly, there are many resources available to make mental health care more affordable and accessible.

Community-based mental health organizations, sliding-scale clinics, and online therapy platforms have made therapy more affordable for individuals who may not have insurance or who cannot afford private therapy. Additionally, many employers offer Employee Assistance Programs (EAPs) that provide free or low-cost counseling services to employees and their families. By raising awareness of these resources, we can break down the myth that therapy is out of reach for those who need it most.

## The Positive Impacts of Mental Health Treatment

Dispelling myths about therapy is only part of the process; it is equally important to highlight the positive impacts of mental health treatment. Therapy has been shown to be an effective tool for improving emotional well-being, reducing symptoms of anxiety and depression, and increasing overall quality of life. Research has consistently shown that therapy can help individuals develop healthier coping mechanisms, improve relationships, and gain greater insight into their thoughts and behaviors.

For Black individuals, therapy can also be a powerful tool for healing from the effects of systemic racism, generational trauma, and cultural stressors. Therapy provides a space to process these experiences, to build resilience, and to develop strategies for navigating the challenges of being Black in a racially biased society.

## Stories of Transformation Through Therapy

One of the most compelling ways to rewrite the narrative around therapy is by sharing stories of transformation. These stories can serve as powerful reminders that seeking help is not only courageous but also life-changing.

1. **Nicole's Story: Overcoming Anxiety Through Therapy** Nicole, a Black woman in her 40s, had always been the "strong one" in her family. She juggled a demanding career, took care of her aging parents, and

supported her younger siblings. But beneath the surface, she was struggling with severe anxiety. After years of trying to manage it on her own, Nicole decided to seek therapy. Through cognitive-behavioral therapy (CBT), she learned how to manage her anxiety, set boundaries, and prioritize her self-care. Nicole now speaks openly about her experience with therapy, encouraging others to seek help when they need it.

2. **Devin's Story: Healing from Childhood Trauma** Devin, a Black man in his early 30s, grew up in a household where emotions were never discussed. As a child, he experienced trauma that he carried into adulthood. Despite his success in his career, Devin found himself struggling with feelings of anger and sadness that he couldn't explain. After a close friend recommended therapy, Devin began working with a Black therapist who specialized in trauma. Through therapy, Devin was able to process his childhood experiences, heal from his trauma, and develop healthier ways of expressing his emotions.

3. **Mariah's Story: Balancing Faith and Therapy** Mariah, a deeply religious Black woman, was hesitant to seek therapy because she believed that her faith should be enough to get her through her struggles with depression. However, after a period of worsening symptoms, Mariah decided to try

faith-based therapy. Her therapist helped her integrate her spiritual practices into her mental health treatment, allowing her to use both prayer and therapeutic techniques to manage her depression. Mariah now sees therapy as a complement to her faith, rather than a contradiction of it.

## Conclusion

Rewriting the narrative around mental health in Black households requires challenging long-held myths and redefining what it means to be strong. Vulnerability, far from being a sign of weakness, is an essential part of emotional well-being and personal growth. Therapy, rather than being a last resort or a sign of failure, is a proactive tool for healing, empowerment, and resilience.

By dispelling the myths that surround therapy and highlighting the positive impacts of mental health treatment, we can encourage more Black individuals and families to seek the help they need. Therapy is not just for the weak—it is for anyone who wants to thrive emotionally, mentally, and spiritually. As we continue to rewrite the narrative, we create a new legacy of strength—one that includes vulnerability, self-awareness, and a commitment to mental health.

# Chapter 4: Starting the Conversation in Black Households

Mental health remains a sensitive and often stigmatized subject in many Black households. For generations, conversations about mental health, therapy, and emotional struggles have either been met with silence or brushed off with well-meaning but dismissive phrases like "pray on it" or "toughen up." However, starting the conversation about mental health, particularly therapy, is an essential step toward breaking the cycle of emotional suppression and encouraging healing. This chapter will provide practical guidance on how to approach these delicate conversations, especially with older generations who may be more resistant to discussing mental health, and offer strategies for using non-judgmental, supportive language that fosters open dialogue instead of defensive reactions.

# Talking to Family: Approaching Mental Health Conversations with Care

## Understanding Generational Perspectives

Before initiating a conversation about mental health and therapy with family members, it is essential to recognize that attitudes toward mental health may differ across generations. Older generations of Black families often grew up during times when discussing mental health was taboo or considered a luxury that only white or affluent people could afford. Their approach to mental health was often shaped by the need to survive in a society that was actively hostile to Black lives. In this context, emotional suppression was seen as a necessary survival tool, and seeking therapy may have been viewed as either unnecessary or a sign of weakness.

For many elders in Black households, mental health challenges were met with resilience, faith, and a strong sense of self-reliance. The idea of sharing one's personal struggles with a therapist—someone outside the family—may be foreign and uncomfortable for them. Understanding these perspectives is crucial when approaching older generations, as it can help you frame the conversation in a way that acknowledges their lived experiences while introducing the idea of therapy as a form of modern self-care.

## Starting with Empathy

The first step in starting a conversation about therapy is to approach the topic with empathy and understanding. Rather than confronting a family member or criticizing their perspective on mental health, it is more effective to acknowledge the challenges they have faced and the ways in which they have learned to cope with life's difficulties. By validating their experiences, you can create a sense of mutual respect and openness.

For example, if you are talking to a grandparent or elder, you might say something like:

*"I've always admired how strong you are and how much you've overcome in your life. I know that things weren't easy growing up, and you've always been there for the family. I wanted to talk about something that I think could be helpful for all of us, especially when we're dealing with stress or emotional struggles."*

This approach shows respect for their life experiences and introduces the idea of therapy in a non-confrontational way. It also opens the door to discussing therapy as a tool that could complement the strength and resilience they already possess, rather than undermining it.

# Framing Therapy as Self-Care, Not a Sign of Weakness

Another important consideration when talking to family members about therapy is to frame it as a form of self-care rather than as a response to failure or weakness. Many people, particularly older generations, still hold the belief that therapy is only for people who are "broken" or who can't handle life on their own. Reframing therapy as a proactive form of self-care can help dispel this misconception.

You might say something like:

*"I've been learning more about how important it is to take care of our mental health, just like we take care of our physical health. Therapy is really just a way to talk through things with someone who's trained to help us understand our emotions and manage stress. It's not about being weak—it's about staying strong and healthy."*

By comparing therapy to taking care of physical health, you can normalize the idea of seeking help and make it clear that therapy is not just for people in crisis but for anyone who wants to improve their emotional well-being. This framing helps to remove the stigma and encourages family members to see therapy as a positive step.

## Introducing the Idea Gradually

For many families, particularly those with older generations, the idea of therapy may be met with initial resistance. It's important to recognize that changing deeply ingrained beliefs about mental health can take time. Rather than expecting immediate acceptance, consider introducing the idea of therapy gradually.

Start by talking about stress, anxiety, or emotional challenges in a general sense. You might share your own experiences with therapy, or talk about a friend or public figure who has benefited from therapy, as a way of showing that it's a common and acceptable practice. Over time, these conversations can help normalize the idea of therapy and make family members more open to considering it for themselves.

For example, you might say:

*"I was talking to a friend the other day who started therapy, and she said it's really helped her with stress. I've been thinking about it too, because I feel like it could be helpful for me to talk through some things I've been feeling."*

By presenting therapy as something that's already being used by people in your social circle, you can make it feel more relatable and less intimidating for family members.

# Offering to Explore Therapy Together

In some cases, family members may be more open to the idea of therapy if they feel supported in the process. Offering to explore therapy together can be a way to ease their concerns and show that they're not alone in this journey. Whether it's attending family therapy sessions together or helping them find a therapist, your support can make a big difference in how receptive they are to the idea.

You might say:

*"I know that talking about mental health can be hard, but I think it could be really helpful for us to explore therapy as a family. I'd be happy to go with you to a session, or we could even try finding a therapist together. It's just something I think could help us all feel more connected and less stressed."*

This approach emphasizes the collective benefits of therapy and frames it as something the family can do together, rather than as an individual burden. It also shows that you are invested in their well-being and willing to take steps to support them.

# Language Matters: How to Discuss Therapy Without Judgment

One of the most important aspects of starting conversations about mental health in Black households is using language that is non-judgmental and supportive. The words we choose can either open the door to meaningful dialogue or shut it down before it even begins. Using language that avoids blame or judgment can help family members feel more comfortable discussing their feelings and considering therapy as an option.

## Avoiding Judgmental Phrases

When talking to family members about therapy, it's important to avoid using phrases that might make them feel defensive or judged. For example, saying things like "You need therapy" or "You've got issues" can come across as accusatory and may cause the person to shut down the conversation.

Instead, try using language that is more supportive and empathetic. For example, you might say:

*"I've noticed that things seem really stressful for you lately, and I just want to make sure you're*

*okay. Sometimes talking to someone can really help."*

By focusing on their well-being rather than diagnosing or criticizing them, you create a space where they feel supported rather than attacked.

## Using "I" Statements

When discussing therapy, it's helpful to use "I" statements rather than "you" statements. "You" statements can make the other person feel blamed or targeted, while "I" statements emphasize your own feelings and concerns in a way that is less confrontational.

For example, instead of saying:

*"You've been really irritable lately, and I think you need to talk to someone."*

You might say:

*"I've been feeling concerned because I've noticed that things have been tough lately. I just want to make sure we're both taking care of our mental health."*

This approach shifts the focus to your own feelings and desires, making the conversation feel more collaborative and less accusatory.

# Emphasizing the Benefits of Therapy

Rather than focusing on what's "wrong" or what needs to be "fixed," try to emphasize the positive benefits of therapy. Talk about how therapy can help improve communication, reduce stress, and strengthen relationships. By highlighting the potential for growth and healing, you can make therapy feel like a hopeful and empowering option rather than a punishment.

For example, you might say:

*"I've been thinking a lot about how we could improve our communication and make sure we're supporting each other. Therapy could be a really good way for us to learn new tools and take care of our mental health together."*

This approach emphasizes the collaborative and constructive nature of therapy, making it feel like a positive step forward rather than a last resort.

# Normalizing Therapy

One of the best ways to encourage open dialogue about therapy is to normalize it as a regular part of life. The more we talk about therapy in casual, non-judgmental terms, the more comfortable family members will feel discussing it. Share your own experiences with therapy, if you have them, or talk about how therapy has helped people you know. The goal is to make therapy feel like a normal, accessible option for everyone.

You might say:

*"I've been hearing more and more about how helpful therapy can be, and I think it's something we should all consider, just like we go to the doctor for checkups. It's a way to take care of our emotional health."*

By normalizing therapy, you help remove the stigma and make it feel like a natural part of maintaining overall well-being.

## Encouraging Open Dialogue

Finally, it's important to create an environment where family members feel safe discussing their feelings and concerns about therapy without fear of judgment. Encourage open dialogue by asking questions and listening actively to their responses. You might ask:

*"What do you think about therapy? Have you ever thought about trying it?"*

By asking open-ended questions, you give your family members the opportunity to share their thoughts and feelings, which can lead to a more productive and meaningful conversation.

## Handling Resistance with Compassion

It's important to recognize that even with the best intentions, some family members may still resist the idea of therapy. If this happens, it's essential to remain compassionate and avoid pushing too hard. Forcing the issue can lead to defensiveness and further resistance. Instead, acknowledge their concerns and let them know that you are there to support them, no matter what.

You might say:

*"I understand if you're not ready to try therapy right now, but I just want you to know that I'm here for you. Whenever you're ready to talk, I'm here to listen."*

This approach keeps the door open for future conversations and shows that you respect their autonomy while still offering your support.

## Conclusion

Starting the conversation about mental health and therapy in Black households is not always easy, but it is a crucial step toward healing and emotional well-being. By approaching these conversations with empathy, using non-judgmental language, and offering support, we can create a space where family members feel comfortable discussing their feelings and considering therapy as a positive option. As we continue to normalize mental health care and break down the stigma surrounding therapy, we can foster a culture of open dialogue, emotional health, and support within our families.

# Chapter 5: The Role of Parents and Guardians

Parents and guardians play a crucial role in shaping the mental health of their children. From the way emotional struggles are handled to the conversations surrounding mental well-being, the foundation for how children approach their mental health is largely built at home. In Black households, where cultural and societal norms have historically stigmatized therapy, parents and guardians have a unique opportunity to break cycles of silence and prioritize emotional health for the next generation. This chapter will focus on how parents can normalize therapy for children and adolescents, and the importance of sharing personal stories to create an open, supportive environment that fosters emotional well-being.

# Normalizing Therapy for Children and Adolescents

## The Importance of Prioritizing Mental Health for Children

Children and adolescents are particularly vulnerable to the stresses of life, whether it's navigating school pressures, managing relationships with peers, or coping with societal expectations. For Black children, additional stressors such as systemic racism, microaggressions, and discrimination add another layer of emotional burden. As a result, mental health care is essential for children and adolescents, who may not yet have the tools to understand or manage these challenges on their own. By normalizing therapy early on, parents and guardians can equip their children with lifelong coping skills and emotional intelligence.

Historically, mental health in Black families has often been addressed reactively—when issues reach a breaking point—rather than proactively. Parents may not seek professional help for their children until they notice significant behavioral changes, such as poor academic performance, social withdrawal, or expressions of anxiety or depression. However, by making mental health a regular part of family conversations and de-stigmatizing therapy, parents can lay the groundwork for their children to view therapy as a positive, proactive tool rather than a last resort.

Therapy for children can help them process their emotions in a healthy way, build self-awareness, and develop resilience. These early interventions can have long-lasting effects, teaching children how to navigate emotional challenges before they escalate into more significant problems. By prioritizing mental health care for their children, parents not only support their immediate well-being but also prepare them for the emotional complexities of adulthood.

## The Long-Term Benefits of Normalizing Therapy Early

One of the most important gifts parents and guardians can give their children is the ability to understand and express their emotions. Therapy provides children and adolescents with the language and tools they need to articulate their feelings, which can prevent emotional bottling and reduce the risk of future mental health crises.

Normalizing therapy early also helps children develop a mindset that seeking help is not only acceptable but encouraged. When therapy is presented as a normal part of life—just like going to the doctor or the dentist—it becomes less intimidating and more accessible. Children who grow up with this mindset are more likely to seek help when they need it, whether during childhood, adolescence, or adulthood.

In addition to providing emotional tools, early therapy interventions can also help children build stronger social relationships. Therapy teaches children how to communicate their needs, set boundaries, and develop empathy for others. These skills are critical for forming healthy relationships with peers, family members, and later, romantic partners. By prioritizing mental health early, parents help their children cultivate the emotional intelligence needed to navigate the complexities of relationships throughout life.

## How Parents Can Normalize Therapy for Their Children

1. **Start with Age-Appropriate Conversations**

   Normalizing therapy for children begins with open, age-appropriate conversations about emotions and mental health. From an early age, parents can introduce the idea that it's okay to feel sad, angry, or frustrated and that these emotions are a normal part of life. By talking about feelings openly, parents can help children understand that mental health is just as important as physical health.

   For younger children, you might say something like:

   *"Sometimes we all feel sad or upset, and that's okay. When we feel that way, it can help to talk to someone about it. That's what therapy is—talking to someone who can*

*help us understand our feelings."*
For older children or teenagers, you can be more specific:
*"Life can be stressful, especially with everything going on at school and in the world. If you ever feel like things are getting too overwhelming, talking to a therapist can help you manage your stress and figure things out."*

2. **Model Emotional Awareness**
   Children learn by watching the adults around them. When parents model emotional awareness and healthy coping strategies, children are more likely to adopt these behaviors. Parents can normalize therapy by being open about their own emotions and how they handle stress. For example, if you're feeling overwhelmed, you might say:
   *"I've had a really tough day, and I'm feeling a little stressed out. I think I'm going to take a break and talk to someone about it, because that helps me feel better."*
   By modeling emotional openness, you show your children that it's okay to talk about feelings and seek help when needed.

3. **Be Open About Therapy as an Option**
   Make therapy a regular part of the conversation when discussing emotional health. When children know that therapy is an option, they are more likely to consider it when they are struggling. You might say:
   *"If you ever feel like things are getting hard,*

*you can always talk to me, and we can figure out if seeing a therapist would help. Therapy is a great way to get extra support when you need it."*

4. **Reduce Stigma by Sharing Positive Stories**

Help break down the stigma surrounding therapy by sharing positive stories of people who have benefited from it. This can include personal stories, stories of friends or family members, or stories from public figures who have openly discussed their mental health journeys. When children see that therapy is a common and helpful tool used by people they respect, they are more likely to view it positively.

5. **Offer Therapy as a Tool, Not a Punishment**

Sometimes, therapy is suggested after a child exhibits challenging behavior, which can lead the child to feel that therapy is a form of punishment. To avoid this, make it clear that therapy is not something to be feared or resented but a tool for understanding and managing emotions. You might say:

*"I know you've been feeling really upset lately, and that's okay. Therapy is something we can try to help you feel better and figure out what's going on. It's not because you're in trouble—it's because I care about you and want to make sure you're okay."*

By framing therapy as a positive resource, parents can help children feel empowered to use it when they need support.

# Breaking the Cycle of Silence: Sharing Personal Stories with Your Kids

## The Importance of Vulnerability in Parenting

For many Black parents and guardians, emotional vulnerability has not always been a comfortable or acceptable part of family life. The cultural emphasis on resilience, strength, and self-reliance has often discouraged parents from sharing their own emotional struggles with their children. However, breaking the cycle of silence around mental health requires a willingness to be open about one's own experiences with emotional challenges, stress, and even therapy.

When parents share their personal stories with their children, they create a safe space for open communication and emotional expression. Children who see their parents model vulnerability are more likely to feel comfortable expressing their own emotions and seeking help when needed. This vulnerability does not mean oversharing or burdening children with adult problems; rather, it means showing them that it's okay to have emotions and that seeking help is a natural part of life.

## How Sharing Personal Stories Can Help Break the Stigma

Sharing personal stories about mental health can help break the stigma surrounding therapy and encourage children to view it as a normal, positive option. When parents talk openly about their own mental health journeys, they humanize the experience of emotional struggle and make it easier for children to relate.

For example, a parent might share a story like this:

*"When I was younger, I used to get really stressed out about work and life, and I didn't always know how to handle it. It wasn't until I talked to someone—a therapist—that I realized it's okay to ask for help. Therapy really helped me understand my feelings and gave me tools to manage stress. That's why I think it's important for you to know that it's okay to talk to someone if you're ever feeling overwhelmed."*

By sharing this type of story, parents show their children that therapy is a useful tool that can help them through difficult times. It also normalizes the idea that everyone faces emotional challenges at some point and that seeking help is a healthy way to cope.

# Encouraging Emotional Expression

One of the most powerful ways parents can support their children's mental health is by encouraging emotional expression. This means creating an environment where children feel safe talking about their feelings without fear of judgment or dismissal. When children know that their emotions will be met with empathy and understanding, they are more likely to open up about their struggles.

Parents can encourage emotional expression by asking open-ended questions and actively listening to their children's responses. For example:

*"How are you feeling today? Is there anything on your mind that you'd like to talk about?"*

*"I noticed you seemed a little upset earlier. Do you want to talk about what's going on?"*

By regularly checking in with their children and creating space for emotional conversations, parents can help their children develop the language and confidence to express their feelings.

# Teaching Emotional Regulation Through Personal Stories

In addition to sharing stories about therapy, parents can also share personal stories about how they manage their emotions in everyday life. For example, a parent might say:

*"Sometimes when I feel really angry or stressed, I take a few deep breaths or go for a walk to calm down. It helps me think more clearly and figure out what I need to do next."*

By sharing these stories, parents teach their children practical emotional regulation skills that they can use in their own lives. These conversations help children understand that emotions are normal and that there are healthy ways to manage them.

## Creating a Safe Space for Dialogue

Sharing personal stories is not just about talking; it's about creating a dialogue where children feel safe to share their own experiences as well. After sharing a personal story, parents can encourage their children to share how they've been feeling or ask if they have any questions about mental health or therapy. By fostering this two-way conversation, parents create an ongoing dialogue about emotional health that can continue as their children grow.

For example, after sharing a story about your own experience with stress, you might ask:

*"Have you ever felt really stressed or overwhelmed? How did you handle it? Do you think talking to someone could help?"*

These questions invite children to reflect on their own experiences and open up about their feelings in a supportive environment.

## The Power of Parental Support

Ultimately, the role of parents and guardians in normalizing therapy and breaking the cycle of silence is rooted in love and support. Children who feel emotionally supported by their parents are more likely to thrive, both mentally and emotionally. By normalizing therapy, sharing personal stories, and encouraging emotional expression, parents can help their children develop a healthy relationship with mental health and set them on a path toward emotional well-being.

## Conclusion

Parents and guardians have a profound impact on how their children perceive and manage their mental health. By normalizing therapy early, parents can equip their children with the tools they need to navigate emotional challenges and develop lifelong emotional intelligence. Sharing personal stories about mental health and therapy can help break the cycle of silence that has often surrounded these topics in Black households, creating a safe space for children to express their feelings and seek help when needed.

As we move forward in rewriting the narrative around mental health, it's clear that parents and guardians are key players in this transformation. By prioritizing mental health, modeling vulnerability, and creating a supportive environment, parents can lay the foundation for a future where therapy is seen not as a last resort but as a powerful tool for growth, healing, and resilience.

# Chapter 6: Black Men and Therapy

The mental health crisis facing Black men is one of the most under-discussed but critical issues in society today. Black men face unique cultural, social, and economic pressures that contribute to high rates of depression, anxiety, and trauma, yet these challenges are often left unspoken due to societal expectations. Chief among these pressures is the enduring stereotype of the "Strong Black man," which reinforces the idea that Black men must be stoic, resilient, and emotionally invulnerable at all times. In this chapter, we will explore the challenges Black men face regarding mental health and therapy, dismantle the "Strong Black man" stereotype, and examine the importance of creating safe spaces where Black men can feel comfortable discussing their emotions.

# Dismantling the "Strong Black Man" Stereotype

## The Origins and Impact of the Stereotype

The "strong Black man" stereotype has roots in both historical and cultural contexts. Historically, during slavery, Black men were often forced to suppress their emotions to survive brutal conditions. Emotional expression, especially vulnerability, was not seen as an option in a world where they were dehumanized and treated as property. Post-slavery, as Black men faced systemic racism, segregation, and violence, stoicism became a form of resilience, a way of coping with an oppressive society that continually sought to diminish their humanity.

Culturally, this expectation of strength has been reinforced over generations. Many Black men grow up hearing phrases like "man up" or "boys don't cry," which communicate that emotional vulnerability is a weakness. Black boys are often socialized to believe that showing emotions like sadness or fear makes them less masculine, and by extension, less valuable. This creates a rigid standard of masculinity that Black men are expected to meet—one that leaves little room for emotional expression or the vulnerability that therapy requires.

The "Strong Black man" stereotype is also perpetuated by media portrayals of Black men as hyper-masculine figures—athletes, entertainers, or figures of physical power—who seem impervious to emotional distress. These depictions reinforce the notion that Black men should not show signs of emotional struggle or ask for help.

## The Harmful Effects of Emotional Suppression

While the "strong Black man" stereotype may seem to celebrate resilience, it actually creates a harmful culture of emotional suppression. When Black men are told that they must always be strong and that seeking help is a sign of weakness, it limits their ability to express their emotions in healthy ways. This emotional repression can lead to:

1. **Mental Health Struggles:** Black men are more likely to experience untreated mental health issues such as depression, anxiety, PTSD, and suicidal thoughts. Studies show that Black men are disproportionately affected by mental health conditions but are less likely to seek therapy than their white counterparts.
2. **Physical Health Issues:** Suppressed emotions can also manifest in physical health problems. Chronic stress, which is linked to conditions like high blood pressure,

heart disease, and stroke, is often a result of unresolved emotional distress. For Black men, who are already at higher risk for these conditions, the added burden of emotional repression can have serious consequences.

3.  **Strained Relationships:** Emotional suppression can make it difficult for Black men to form close, meaningful relationships. Whether in romantic partnerships, friendships, or family dynamics, the inability to express emotions openly can create distance and misunderstanding. This can lead to isolation and loneliness, even in the presence of loved ones.

4.  **Anger and Aggression:** In some cases, the pressure to suppress emotions can lead to outbursts of anger or aggression. When Black men are taught that the only acceptable emotional expression is anger, they may channel their suppressed feelings into aggressive behaviors, which can further perpetuate negative stereotypes about Black men as violent or dangerous.

## The Power of Vulnerability

To dismantle the "Strong Black man" stereotype, it is essential to redefine strength in a way that includes emotional vulnerability. Vulnerability is not a sign of weakness but a courageous act of self-awareness and self-care. It takes strength to acknowledge one's emotions, to seek help, and to prioritize mental health.

In therapy, Black men have the opportunity to explore their emotions in a safe, supportive environment where they are not judged for being vulnerable. Therapy provides a space for Black men to process the stress, trauma, and emotional pain they may have been carrying in silence for years. By breaking the cycle of emotional suppression, therapy empowers Black men to heal and redefine what it means to be strong.

Redefining strength in vulnerability means challenging the belief that Black men must always "have it together." It means acknowledging that everyone, regardless of gender or race, experiences emotional struggles and that seeking help is a responsible and healthy choice. When Black men are given permission to express their emotions openly and seek therapy without fear of judgment, they can begin to heal from the pressures of living up to an unrealistic standard of masculinity.

# Creating Safe Spaces for Black Men

## Why Safe Spaces Are Essential for Black Men

One of the biggest barriers to therapy for Black men is the lack of safe spaces where they feel comfortable discussing their mental health. Therapy can feel intimidating for anyone, but for Black men who have been conditioned to suppress their emotions, the idea of opening up to a therapist—especially one who may not share their cultural background or experiences—can feel particularly daunting. That's why creating environments where Black men feel safe to express their emotions, whether within therapy, family, or community spaces, is crucial.

Safe spaces are environments where individuals can speak openly about their feelings and experiences without fear of judgment, discrimination, or shame. For Black men, these spaces are essential for several reasons:

1. **Breaking Down the Fear of Vulnerability:** Safe spaces allow Black men to express vulnerability in a supportive environment. Knowing that they won't be judged for showing emotion or asking for help can encourage Black men to share their struggles and seek solutions.
2. **Culturally Competent Support:** For therapy to be effective, Black men need access to therapists who understand their cultural experiences and the specific challenges they face, such as racism, racial trauma, and societal expectations of masculinity. Culturally competent therapists are more likely to create an environment where Black men feel understood and validated.
3. **Community and Peer Support:** In addition to therapy, peer-led support groups for

Black men can serve as safe spaces for discussing mental health. These groups provide opportunities for Black men to connect with others who share similar experiences and challenges. Seeing other Black men open up about their mental health can be a powerful form of validation and encouragement.

## How to Create Safe Spaces for Black Men in Therapy

Creating safe spaces for Black men in therapy begins with the therapist's approach. Therapists who work with Black men must be intentional about fostering trust and understanding. Here are some key elements that contribute to creating a safe therapeutic environment:

1. **Cultural Competence:** Therapists should be knowledgeable about the cultural, social, and historical factors that impact the mental health of Black men. This includes understanding the effects of systemic racism, racial trauma, and the "strong Black man" stereotype. Therapists who are culturally competent are better equipped to offer support that resonates with their clients' lived experiences.
2. **Active Listening and Non-Judgmental Attitude:** For Black men who have been conditioned to suppress their emotions, therapy can feel like a vulnerable

experience. Therapists should practice active listening and ensure that their clients feel heard and understood without judgment. A non-judgmental attitude allows clients to explore their emotions openly without fear of criticism or invalidation.

3. **Affirming Black Masculinity in All Its Forms:** Part of creating a safe space for Black men is affirming that there is no one way to "be a man." Black men come from diverse backgrounds and experiences, and their expressions of masculinity are equally varied. Therapists should avoid reinforcing stereotypes about masculinity and instead affirm the individuality of each client.

4. **Offering Space for Discussions About Race:** Black men often face unique challenges related to race and racism that affect their mental health. These experiences may not always be acknowledged in therapy, especially if the therapist does not share the same cultural background. Therapists should create space for discussions about race and validate the impact that racism has on their clients' emotional well-being.

5. **Encouraging Emotional Expression Without Pressure:** Many Black men may feel unsure or uncomfortable expressing emotions in therapy, especially if they have been taught to suppress their feelings. Therapists should encourage emotional expression in a way that feels safe and

comfortable for the client, without pressuring them to open up before they are ready. Over time, as trust is built, clients may feel more comfortable sharing their emotions.

# Building Safe Spaces in the Family and Community

Creating safe spaces for Black men is not only the responsibility of therapists but also of families and communities. Black men need environments, both at home and in their social circles, where they feel supported in discussing their mental health. Here's how families and communities can help create these safe spaces:

1. **Normalizing Emotional Conversations in the Family:** Families can play a critical role in normalizing conversations about mental health. Rather than reinforcing the idea that Black men must always be strong, families can create an environment where emotional expression is welcomed and supported. Parents, siblings, and partners can encourage Black men to share their feelings and seek help when needed without fear of judgment.
2. **Peer Support Groups for Black Men:** Community-based support groups can provide Black men with a safe space to discuss their mental health among peers. These groups allow Black men to connect with others who share similar experiences

and challenges, offering both validation and camaraderie. Peer support groups can also reduce the stigma around therapy by showing that it is normal for Black men to seek help.

3. **Mentorship and Role Models:** Positive role models who speak openly about their mental health journeys can have a profound impact on Black men. Public figures, community leaders, or mentors who have sought therapy can help normalize mental health care and encourage others to do the same. Seeing someone they respect talk about therapy can reduce the stigma and make it more acceptable for Black men to seek help.

4. **Creating Spaces for Black Men in Faith Communities:** For many Black men, faith plays a central role in their lives. Churches and religious communities can also serve as safe spaces for discussing mental health. Faith leaders who encourage mental health discussions and promote therapy as a complement to spiritual well-being can help reduce the stigma around therapy in religious settings.

## Conclusion

The challenges Black men face regarding mental health are deeply rooted in cultural expectations, societal pressures, and the long-standing "strong Black man" stereotype. Dismantling this stereotype is essential for creating an environment where Black men can seek therapy and emotional support without fear of judgment or shame. Vulnerability is not a sign of weakness but a courageous act of self-care and healing.

Creating safe spaces—both within therapy and in the family or community—where Black men can openly discuss their mental health is crucial for breaking the cycle of emotional suppression. By fostering these environments, we can empower Black men to embrace their emotions, seek help when needed, and redefine strength in a way that includes mental health and emotional well-being. Through this process, Black men can heal, grow, and thrive.

# Chapter 7: Therapy for the Black Woman

Black women carry a unique set of pressures and expectations rooted in historical and cultural norms. These pressures, often symbolized by the "superwoman complex," demand that Black women be strong, self-reliant, and capable of taking care of everyone else while neglecting their own needs. This societal expectation significantly impacts their mental health and often makes therapy seem like an unnecessary or even shameful act of vulnerability. In this chapter, we will examine how the superwoman complex influences Black women's perceptions of mental health and therapy, and explore the importance of building support systems such as sister circles to supplement therapy and foster collective healing.

# Mental Health and the Superwoman Complex

## The Origins of the Superwoman Complex

The superwoman complex is a cultural phenomenon that places an immense burden on Black women to be strong, resilient, and self-sacrificing. Historically, Black women have been expected to endure emotional, physical, and mental hardships in silence, from the legacy of slavery to the present-day challenges of racism, sexism, and economic inequality. The image of the Black woman as the "superwoman" is deeply ingrained in the collective consciousness, celebrated in popular culture, and reinforced in Black families and communities.

This complex evolved as a survival strategy during times of intense adversity. During slavery, Black women were expected to labor in the fields alongside men, care for their own families, and often serve as caretakers for their oppressors. This multi-layered role, where they bore immense responsibility without the luxury of rest or vulnerability, became a defining characteristic of the Black woman's experience. Over time, this image of the "strong Black woman" persisted, and it became intertwined with notions of dignity, pride, and resilience.

However, while resilience and strength are admirable qualities, the superwoman complex comes at a cost. It leaves little room for Black women to express vulnerability, seek help, or prioritize their own mental health. The pressure to always "hold it together" can lead to burnout, depression, anxiety, and emotional exhaustion. Despite their strength, Black women are often left feeling isolated and unsupported, as they are expected to be the backbone of their families and communities without showing any signs of struggle.

## The Role of Caretaker: Emotional Labor and Mental Health

At the heart of the superwoman complex is the role of caretaker. Black women are often socialized to put the needs of others before their own, whether it's caring for their children, partners, extended families, or even their communities. This expectation is rooted in both cultural and gendered norms, where Black women are seen as the emotional caretakers of those around them. While caretaking can be a source of pride and fulfillment, it also leads to an overwhelming amount of emotional labor that goes unnoticed and unacknowledged.

Emotional labor refers to the work of managing and responding to the emotions of others, often at the expense of one's own emotional well-being. For Black women, this labor often extends into every aspect of their lives. They may feel responsible for the emotional health of their families, ensuring that everyone is taken care of and that conflicts are resolved. They are often expected to remain strong in the face of adversity, managing their own emotions while also absorbing the emotions of others.

This constant caretaking can lead to emotional burnout, where Black women feel drained, exhausted, and unable to take care of themselves. Burnout, combined with the cultural pressure to maintain the appearance of strength, can prevent Black women from seeking therapy or acknowledging their need for help. The superwoman complex convinces many Black women that asking for help is a sign of failure, and that their worth is tied to their ability to manage everything on their own.

## How the Superwoman Complex Impacts Perceptions of Therapy

The superwoman complex has a significant impact on how Black women perceive therapy. In many cases, therapy is seen as something that only "weak" or "unstable" people need, and the idea of seeking professional help may feel incompatible with the image of strength that Black women are expected to embody. Black women may feel that admitting to needing therapy means admitting that they can't handle life's challenges

—a notion that goes against the very core of the superwoman identity.

Additionally, Black women may feel that their emotional struggles will not be taken seriously by others, especially in a society that often devalues Black women's experiences and contributions. The fear of being labeled "dramatic" or "overreacting" can prevent Black women from speaking openly about their mental health needs, even within their own families or communities.

Another factor that contributes to Black women's reluctance to seek therapy is the historical mistrust of medical and mental health institutions. Many Black women have experienced or are aware of the systemic racism within healthcare systems, which often leads to concerns that their experiences will be misunderstood, minimized, or dismissed by therapists who do not share their cultural background. This mistrust, coupled with the superwoman complex, can create a barrier to accessing therapy.

However, therapy offers Black women a space to prioritize their own emotional health, process their experiences, and release the burdens of caretaking. By dismantling the superwoman complex and redefining strength to include vulnerability and self-care, Black women can begin to see therapy not as a weakness but as an act of self-preservation and empowerment.

# Building a Support System: Sister Circles and Therapy

## The Importance of Support Systems

While therapy is an essential tool for mental health, it is not the only form of support that Black women need. In addition to individual therapy, building a strong support system is crucial for fostering emotional well-being. For many Black women, sister circles—collective spaces for healing, sharing, and support—serve as a vital complement to therapy.

A support system provides Black women with a community of people who understand their experiences and can offer empathy, encouragement, and validation. These relationships are particularly important for combating the isolation that often accompanies the superwoman complex. When Black women feel supported by others who share similar challenges, they are more likely to open up about their struggles and seek help when needed.

## What Are Sister Circles?

Sister circles are communal spaces where Black women gather to share their experiences, offer support, and engage in collective healing. These spaces are built on trust, mutual respect, and the understanding that Black women's experiences are unique and deserving of validation. Sister circles can take many forms, from informal gatherings of friends to organized groups focused on mental health, self-care, or personal development.

Historically, Black women have always turned to one another for support in times of need. Whether through church groups, social clubs, or extended family networks, sisterhood has been a powerful source of resilience and empowerment. Today, sister circles continue this tradition by providing Black women with a space where they can be vulnerable, express their emotions, and receive support without fear of judgment.

## How Sister Circles Can Supplement Therapy

While therapy provides an individualized space for processing emotions and addressing mental health issues, sister circles offer collective support that can complement the therapeutic process. Here's how sister circles and therapy can work together to support Black women's mental health:

1. **Validation of Shared Experiences:** In sister circles, Black women have the opportunity to share their experiences and hear from others who have faced similar challenges. This sense of shared experience can be incredibly validating and can help Black women feel less isolated in

their struggles. Therapy, while personalized, can sometimes feel solitary, but sister circles provide a communal aspect of healing that reminds Black women they are not alone.

2. **Emotional Support Between Therapy Sessions:** Therapy sessions typically occur weekly or biweekly, which means that there are periods between sessions when emotional support may be needed. Sister circles offer an ongoing support system that Black women can turn to for encouragement, advice, or simply a listening ear during these in-between times. Having access to both professional support and peer support can create a more comprehensive mental health care system.

3. **Collective Healing Practices:** Many sister circles incorporate collective healing practices such as meditation, journaling, group discussions, and rituals that promote emotional well-being. These practices can supplement the work being done in therapy by providing additional tools for self-care and stress relief. For example, a therapist may recommend journaling as a way to process emotions, and a sister circle may offer guided journaling sessions to support this practice.

4. **Breaking the Silence Together:** The superwoman complex often isolates Black women, making them feel that they must carry their burdens alone. Sister circles

provide a space where Black women can break the silence around their mental health struggles and feel supported by others who understand the pressures they face. By sharing their stories and hearing others do the same, Black women can begin to dismantle the superwoman complex together.

5.  **Encouraging Therapy in a Supportive Environment:** Sister circles can also serve as a space where therapy is normalized and encouraged. When Black women see others in their sister circle seeking therapy and benefiting from it, they may feel more comfortable considering therapy for themselves. Sister circles can help reduce the stigma around therapy by promoting it as a healthy and proactive form of self-care.

# Building and Maintaining a Strong Support System

For Black women, building and maintaining a strong support system is essential for mental health and emotional well-being. In addition to sister circles, Black women can cultivate support networks that include family, friends, mentors, and mental health professionals. Here are some key steps for building a robust support system:

1.  **Identify Safe and Supportive People:** Start by identifying people in your life who make you feel safe, understood, and

supported. These individuals should be people you can turn to when you need emotional support or encouragement. It's important to seek out relationships where you feel comfortable expressing vulnerability without fear of judgment.

2.  **Prioritize Open Communication:** In any support system, open communication is key. Make it a priority to communicate openly and honestly with the people in your support network. Let them know how you're feeling, what you need, and how they can support you. In turn, offer the same level of support to others in your network.

3.  **Set Boundaries for Self-Care:** While having a support system is important, it's also essential to set boundaries that prioritize your own self-care. As Black women often take on the role of caretakers, it can be easy to overextend yourself emotionally. Setting boundaries around your time, energy, and emotional labor ensures that you have the space to care for yourself while also supporting others.

4.  **Join or Start a Sister Circle:** If you don't already have a sister circle, consider joining one or starting your own. Look for community groups, social media forums, or mental health organizations that offer sister circles for Black women. If you prefer to start your own, gather a group of friends or acquaintances who share similar goals for emotional support and healing.

# Conclusion

For Black women, the superwoman complex has long been a source of pride and resilience, but it also places an immense burden on their mental health. The expectation to be strong, self-reliant, and emotionally invulnerable can prevent Black women from seeking therapy or acknowledging their need for help. By dismantling the superwoman complex and redefining strength to include vulnerability, Black women can begin to prioritize their own mental health and embrace therapy as a powerful tool for healing.

In addition to therapy, sister circles and other collective healing spaces provide Black women with the support and validation they need to navigate life's challenges. These spaces offer a sense of community, shared experience, and emotional support that can supplement the work being done in therapy. By building strong support systems and creating environments where therapy is normalized and encouraged, Black women can break the cycle of emotional isolation and embrace mental health as a vital part of their well-being.

# Chapter 8: Finding Culturally Competent Therapists

Culturally competent therapy is an essential element in the mental health care journey, particularly for Black individuals and families. Therapy is most effective when clients feel understood, respected, and safe enough to express their emotions without fear of judgment or misunderstanding. For Black individuals, who often face unique cultural dynamics, racial stress, and generational trauma, finding a therapist who understands these experiences is crucial to creating an environment of healing. In this chapter, we will explore why culturally relevant therapy matters, how it enhances the therapeutic process, and provide resources for finding Black or culturally competent therapists.

# Why Culturally Relevant Therapy Matters

## Understanding the Black Experience

The importance of culturally competent therapy cannot be overstated. For many Black individuals, traditional therapy may feel disconnected from their lived experiences due to differences in cultural understanding, communication styles, or the failure to address the systemic and racial factors that impact their mental health. Culturally competent therapists are trained to understand the historical and cultural context that shapes the emotional and psychological experiences of their clients. They acknowledge and validate the impact of racism, discrimination, and cultural expectations on mental health, which is essential for effective treatment.

For Black families, therapy sessions that fail to take into account the unique cultural pressures—such as the expectations of strength, the legacy of generational trauma, and the challenges of navigating predominantly white spaces—can lead to misunderstandings or a lack of trust. Black clients may feel that their experiences are being minimized or misunderstood if their therapist is not culturally informed. In contrast, culturally competent therapists are more likely to approach therapy with sensitivity to the specific struggles their clients face, fostering a deeper connection and more effective therapeutic outcomes.

# Addressing Systemic Racism and Racial Trauma

One of the key challenges that Black individuals face in therapy is the impact of racial trauma and systemic racism. Racial trauma refers to the psychological and emotional harm caused by repeated exposure to racism, discrimination, and microaggressions. This trauma can manifest as anxiety, depression, hypervigilance, or feelings of worthlessness, all of which are exacerbated by living in a society that devalues Black lives.

Culturally competent therapists are aware of the pervasive effects of racial trauma and know how to address these issues in therapy. They can provide a safe space for clients to process the emotional impact of racism and help them develop coping strategies for dealing with racial stress. For Black clients, knowing that their therapist understands the realities of systemic racism and how it affects mental health can be a huge relief. It allows them to discuss their experiences openly without having to explain or defend their feelings, which is often an added burden in therapy sessions with culturally uninformed therapists.

Therapists who are not culturally competent may overlook or fail to address the role that racism plays in their client's mental health, potentially leaving significant issues unresolved. In contrast, culturally relevant therapy acknowledges these experiences, making it easier for clients to heal from the trauma and stress of navigating a racially biased world.

## Building Trust and Reducing Stigma

For many Black individuals, mistrust of the healthcare system, including mental health services, stems from a long history of medical racism and exploitation. Incidents like the Tuskegee Syphilis Study, forced sterilization of Black women, and ongoing disparities in healthcare access and treatment have contributed to this mistrust. As a result, many Black individuals are hesitant to engage with therapists or other healthcare professionals, fearing that they will not be treated with respect or fairness.

Culturally competent therapists can help reduce this mistrust by creating a therapeutic environment that is respectful, validating, and empowering. When Black clients feel that their therapist understands their cultural background and values, they are more likely to engage in therapy and trust the process. This trust is critical for the therapeutic relationship, as it allows clients to feel comfortable opening up about their emotions and challenges.

Additionally, culturally relevant therapy can help reduce the stigma surrounding mental health in Black communities. When Black clients work with therapists who understand their cultural dynamics, they are more likely to view therapy as a positive and affirming experience. This can lead to a broader acceptance of therapy within Black families and communities, breaking down the stigma that often surrounds mental health care.

# Where to Start: Resources for Finding Black or Culturally Competent Therapists

Finding a culturally competent therapist can seem daunting, especially for individuals who are new to therapy or unsure of where to look. However, there are several resources available that can help families find therapists who are not only licensed and qualified but also understand and respect the cultural dynamics of Black clients. Here are some key places to start:

## 1. Therapy for Black Girls

**Therapy for Black Girls** is a popular online directory and resource dedicated to helping Black women find culturally competent mental health care. The platform was created by Dr. Joy Harden Bradford, a licensed psychologist, with the goal of creating a space where Black women can access therapists who understand their unique needs and experiences. The directory allows users to search for Black female therapists across the United States, providing detailed information about each therapist's background, specialties, and approach to care.

In addition to the directory, Therapy for Black Girls offers a wealth of resources, including blog posts, podcasts, and discussion forums, all focused on promoting mental health and wellness in Black communities. This platform is a valuable starting point for Black women seeking therapy from someone who shares their cultural background and can provide culturally relevant support.

**Website**: therapyforblackgirls.com

## 2. Therapy for Black Men

Similar to Therapy for Black Girls, **Therapy for Black Men** is an online platform designed to connect Black men with culturally competent therapists. The site was created in response to the specific mental health challenges Black men face, including the pressures of masculinity, racial trauma, and the stigma surrounding therapy. Therapy for Black Men features a directory of Black male therapists who specialize in working with Black men and their unique emotional and psychological needs.

In addition to the directory, the platform offers resources aimed at normalizing therapy for Black men and encouraging them to seek help when needed. By providing a space where Black men can find therapists who understand their experiences, Therapy for Black Men helps break down the barriers to mental health care and fosters a culture of emotional wellness.

**Website**: therapyforblackmen.org

# 3. National Queer and Trans Therapists of Color Network (NQTTCN)

For Black individuals who identify as LGBTQ+, the **National Queer and Trans Therapists of Color Network (NQTTCN)** is an essential resource. This network is dedicated to increasing access to mental health care for queer and trans people of color, including Black individuals. The directory includes therapists who specialize in working with queer and trans clients of color, providing culturally competent and affirming care.

NQTTCN offers a space where individuals can find therapists who understand the intersectionality of race, gender, and sexual orientation, ensuring that clients receive care that addresses all aspects of their identity. This resource is particularly valuable for Black LGBTQ+ individuals who may face additional challenges in finding therapists who are both culturally competent and affirming of their gender and sexual identities.

**Website**: nqttcn.com

# 4. Inclusive Therapists

**Inclusive Therapists** is a directory designed to make mental health care accessible to people from marginalized communities, including Black individuals, people of color, LGBTQ+ individuals, and those with disabilities. The platform is committed to promoting equity, justice, and cultural humility in therapy, offering a directory of therapists who are trained in providing culturally competent and inclusive care.

Users can search for therapists based on a variety of criteria, including race, gender, and specialization, making it easier to find a therapist who meets their specific needs. Inclusive Therapists also offers a sliding-scale fee option for clients who may face financial barriers to accessing therapy.

**Website**: inclusivetherapists.com

# 5. Open Path Collective

For individuals and families seeking affordable mental health care, **Open Path Collective** offers a directory of therapists who provide therapy at reduced rates. Many of the therapists listed on Open Path are culturally competent and have experience working with Black clients and communities of color. This platform is particularly helpful for individuals who may not have insurance or who need to find a therapist with sliding-scale fees.

While Open Path Collective is not exclusively for Black individuals, it provides a valuable resource for finding therapists who offer accessible, affordable care.

**Website**: openpathcollective.org

## 6. Psychology Today

**Psychology Today** is one of the largest online directories for finding licensed therapists. While it is not specific to Black therapists or culturally competent care, Psychology Today allows users to search for therapists based on race, specialization, and other factors. Many therapists on the platform include detailed profiles outlining their experience and approach to therapy, making it easier for clients to find culturally competent therapists who understand their needs.

When searching for a therapist on Psychology Today, it's helpful to filter by race or ethnicity to find Black therapists or therapists who specialize in working with Black clients.

**Website**: psychologytoday.com

# 7. Therapy Den

**Therapy Den** is an inclusive directory of therapists that allows users to search based on a variety of criteria, including race, gender, and specialization. Therapy Den is committed to promoting diversity and inclusion in mental health care, offering a platform where individuals can find therapists who are culturally competent and aligned with their specific needs.

The directory includes therapists who specialize in working with Black clients, people of color, LGBTQ+ individuals, and those from other marginalized communities. Therapy Den is a valuable resource for finding therapists who prioritize social justice, equity, and culturally relevant care.

**Website**: therapyden.com

# 8. BetterHelp

**BetterHelp** is a popular online therapy platform that connects clients with licensed therapists through video, phone, or messaging sessions. BetterHelp provides a flexible, convenient option for those seeking therapy, especially for individuals who may have busy schedules or limited access to in-person therapists. The platform offers a diverse pool of therapists, including many who specialize in working with Black individuals and people of color. Users can filter for therapists based on their specific preferences, including cultural competence and areas of expertise.

While BetterHelp is not exclusively for Black clients, it allows for easy matching with therapists who understand the unique cultural and social challenges faced by Black individuals. The platform's convenience and accessibility make it a great option for those seeking therapy from the comfort of their home.

**Website**: betterhelp.com

# Conclusion

Culturally competent therapy is an essential aspect of effective mental health care for Black individuals and families. Finding a therapist who understands and respects the cultural dynamics of Black clients can enhance the therapeutic process by fostering trust, validating lived experiences, and addressing the unique challenges that Black individuals face. By seeking out culturally relevant therapy, Black clients can engage in a healing process that acknowledges their full identity and experiences, leading to more meaningful and lasting emotional well-being.

The resources provided in this chapter offer a starting point for families and individuals to find Black or culturally competent therapists who can connect with their specific needs and values. Whether through directories like Therapy for Black Girls and Therapy for Black Men, or broader platforms like Inclusive Therapists and Psychology Today, there are many options available for finding a therapist who can provide the culturally relevant care that Black individuals deserve.

# Chapter 9: Media, Representation, and Mental Health

The media plays a powerful role in shaping cultural attitudes and narratives, including those surrounding mental health. For Black individuals and communities, media representation has been both a source of empowerment and a site of harmful stereotypes and misconceptions. The way Black people are portrayed in movies, television, music, and social media can deeply influence how mental health and therapy are perceived within Black households. This chapter will explore how media representation impacts Black mental health narratives and discuss the importance of creating new, positive narratives in media and pop culture. We will also showcase Black celebrities, influencers, and media figures who have embraced therapy and are helping to normalize conversations around mental health in the Black community.

# The Impact of Media on Black Mental Health Narratives

## Negative Representations and Their Consequences

Historically, Black people in media have often been portrayed in one-dimensional roles that reinforce harmful stereotypes. These depictions can have a profound impact on the mental health of Black audiences, as they shape how individuals view themselves and how society views them. The media has frequently portrayed Black people as either overly resilient, violent, or emotionally detached—representations that limit the visibility of their emotional complexity and humanity.

1. **The "Strong Black Woman" Stereotype**
   The media frequently upholds the "strong Black woman" stereotype, which celebrates Black women as resilient and unbreakable but often at the expense of their mental well-being. This portrayal reinforces the idea that Black women should not show vulnerability or seek help, perpetuating the superwoman complex discussed in earlier chapters. While strength and resilience are important qualities, the constant depiction of Black women as self-sacrificing and emotionally invulnerable discourages them from addressing their own mental health

needs and can lead to emotional burnout and isolation.

2. **The "Angry Black Man" Stereotype**
Black men are often depicted in the media as aggressive, violent, or emotionally unavailable. This portrayal reinforces the stereotype that Black men are not allowed to be vulnerable or express their emotions, particularly sadness, fear, or anxiety. The "angry Black man" trope not only dehumanizes Black men but also creates a cultural expectation that they must suppress their emotions, making it harder for them to seek therapy or talk openly about their mental health struggles.

3. **Pathologizing Black Lives**
In some media representations, the struggles of Black people are reduced to pathology. This is especially prevalent in stories that center on poverty, crime, and trauma without acknowledging the systemic factors that contribute to these conditions. These portrayals often ignore the broader context of systemic racism and oppression, instead framing mental health challenges as inherent to Black people. This pathologization stigmatizes mental health issues and discourages Black people from seeking help, as they may internalize the idea that their struggles are inevitable or that therapy cannot offer meaningful solutions.

# Positive Representations and Their Benefits

While negative portrayals of Black mental health in media have been pervasive, there has been a significant shift in recent years toward more positive and nuanced representations. These portrayals offer counter-narratives that highlight the emotional complexity of Black characters and emphasize the importance of mental health care.

1. **Representation of Therapy in Black Narratives**
   In television shows, films, and documentaries, we are seeing more Black characters and real-life figures openly discussing mental health and seeking therapy. These representations help to normalize therapy as a valid and necessary tool for emotional well-being. When Black characters are shown attending therapy sessions or working through emotional struggles in a realistic and compassionate manner, it sends the message that mental health care is for everyone, including Black individuals and families.

2. **Challenging Stereotypes**
   Positive media representations challenge harmful stereotypes by portraying Black people as fully realized individuals with a wide range of emotions. Rather than reinforcing the idea that Black people must always be strong or detached, these

representations allow for vulnerability, emotional growth, and healing. For example, shows like *Insecure* and *Queen Sugar* depict Black characters dealing with complex emotions, trauma, and mental health struggles while also showing them seeking support through therapy, friendships, and community.

3.  **Empowerment Through Authenticity** Positive media representations can empower Black viewers by validating their experiences and showing that they are not alone in their struggles. Seeing characters or public figures who look like them navigating mental health issues in relatable ways can encourage Black individuals to take their own mental health seriously. This visibility can break down the stigma around mental health and therapy, particularly for those who have been taught that seeking help is a sign of weakness.

# Creating New Narratives in Media and Pop Culture

## The Power of Black Celebrities and Influencers

In recent years, many Black celebrities, influencers, and public figures have used their platforms to openly discuss mental health and therapy. These individuals play a crucial role in creating new narratives around mental health by normalizing therapy, reducing stigma, and encouraging their fans and followers to prioritize their emotional well-being. The influence of these figures cannot be underestimated—when public figures speak openly about their mental health journeys, they give permission for others to do the same.

Here are some Black celebrities and influencers who have embraced therapy and are helping to shift the narrative around mental health in the Black community:

1.  **Taraji P. Henson**
    Award-winning actress Taraji P. Henson has been an outspoken advocate for mental health in the Black community. After facing her own mental health challenges following the death of her father and the pressures of her career, Henson founded the Boris Lawrence Henson Foundation, named after her father, to address mental health issues in Black communities. The foundation works to provide mental health resources and services, and Henson regularly uses her platform to speak about the importance of therapy and emotional well-being.
2.  **Charlamagne Tha God**
    Radio host and author Charlamagne Tha God has been vocal about his struggles with anxiety and the importance of seeking therapy. In his book *Shook One: Anxiety Playing Tricks on Me*, Charlamagne

candidly discusses his experiences with mental health and how therapy has helped him manage his anxiety. By being open about his own therapy journey, he encourages Black men to prioritize their mental health and break free from the stigma that often surrounds therapy in the Black community.

3. **Gabrielle Union**

Actress and activist Gabrielle Union has been a strong advocate for mental health, particularly around issues of trauma, anxiety, and PTSD. Union has spoken publicly about her experiences with therapy following her experiences of sexual assault and infertility, emphasizing that seeking help has been crucial to her healing process. By sharing her story, Union is helping to break down barriers around mental health care for Black women and normalizing therapy as an essential part of self-care.

4. **Michelle Obama**

Former First Lady Michelle Obama has also been a powerful voice for mental health awareness. In her podcast and book *Becoming*, she discusses the pressures of public life, the importance of therapy, and how she prioritizes her mental health in the face of stress and scrutiny. Her candid discussions about mental health, combined with her influence, have helped open up important conversations about therapy in the Black community.

5. **DeMar DeRozan and Kevin Love**
   In the world of sports, NBA players DeMar DeRozan and Kevin Love have made waves by speaking openly about their struggles with mental health. DeRozan, a Black athlete, shared his experiences with depression and anxiety, challenging the stereotype that Black men, especially in sports, must always appear strong and emotionless. His openness helped pave the way for others in the sports world to speak out about mental health, showing that therapy is an important tool for athletes as well as everyday people.

## Media Platforms Supporting Mental Health Conversations

In addition to celebrities, there are various media platforms that have taken on the responsibility of promoting mental health conversations in the Black community. These platforms play a critical role in creating a space for open dialogue and providing resources for those seeking mental health support.

1. **Podcasts**
   Podcasts like *The Friend Zone*, *Therapy for Black Girls*, and *Black Mental Health Matters* focus on mental health topics relevant to Black listeners. These podcasts offer insights, advice, and personal stories from hosts and guests, helping to normalize

therapy and provide practical mental health tips. The casual, conversational format makes mental health discussions more accessible and relatable for listeners, encouraging them to seek help if needed.

2. **Documentaries**

   Documentaries like *The Me You Can't See* (co-produced by Oprah Winfrey and Prince Harry) and *A Conversation About Mental Health in Black America* offer in-depth explorations of mental health issues in Black communities. These documentaries often feature interviews with Black public figures and everyday individuals who share their mental health journeys, providing a platform for visibility and education. Documentaries are a powerful tool for changing the narrative around mental health, as they provide real-world examples of healing and recovery.

3. **Social Media Campaigns**

   Social media has also become a powerful platform for mental health advocacy in the Black community. Hashtags like #BlackMentalHealthMatters, #YouGoodMan, and #TherapyForBlackGirls create spaces for Black individuals to share their experiences with therapy, offer support to one another, and connect with mental health resources. Influencers, therapists, and activists use platforms like Instagram, Twitter, and YouTube to raise awareness about mental health issues, encourage therapy, and provide educational content tailored to Black audiences.

## The Future of Mental Health Representation in Media

While significant progress has been made in how mental health is portrayed in the media, there is still much work to be done. Moving forward, media creators, producers, and influencers must continue to prioritize authentic and diverse representations of Black mental health. This includes telling stories that reflect the full emotional range of Black people, breaking down stereotypes, and showcasing therapy as a positive, normal part of life.

By creating media that highlights the importance of mental health and therapy, we can continue to shift the narrative in Black communities. The more we see Black people prioritizing their mental health on screen, in music, and in public life, the more normalized it will become in Black households, leading to healthier individuals, families, and communities.

# Conclusion

Media representation plays a powerful role in shaping how Black individuals and communities perceive mental health and therapy. While harmful stereotypes have long dominated media portrayals, the growing presence of positive, nuanced representations is helping to change the narrative. By challenging the "strong Black woman" and "angry Black man" stereotypes and highlighting the value of therapy, the media can serve as a tool for normalizing mental health care in Black households.

Black celebrities, influencers, and media figures who have embraced therapy and spoken openly about their mental health journeys are paving the way for others to do the same. Their visibility helps to break down the stigma surrounding therapy and encourages Black individuals to seek the help they need. As we continue to create and support new narratives in media and pop culture, we can foster a culture of emotional well-being and mental health care in Black communities.

# Chapter 10: Schools, Community Centers, and Churches: Partnering for Mental Health

Mental health challenges often go unaddressed in Black households due to cultural stigma, lack of access, and mistrust of mental health institutions. However, schools, community centers, and churches—the pillars of many Black communities—hold immense potential for transforming attitudes toward mental health. By working together, these institutions can help initiate conversations, provide mental health education, and create safe spaces for seeking therapy. This chapter will explore the role of schools in mental health advocacy, particularly for Black youth, and discuss how churches and community centers can become safe havens that destigmatize therapy and support mental wellness in Black communities.

# The Role of Schools in Mental Health Advocacy

## Schools as Gateways to Mental Health Conversations

Schools are often the first institutional touchpoint for children and adolescents outside of the family. They play a vital role in shaping young minds, fostering emotional growth, and providing support systems. Given the amount of time children spend in school, educational institutions have the power to significantly influence mental health awareness and advocacy, especially for Black youth.

For many Black students, mental health challenges may arise as a result of a variety of factors—academic pressure, social dynamics, discrimination, bullying, or the stress of navigating a predominantly white institution. In some cases, racial trauma and microaggressions experienced in school settings can negatively impact students' mental well-being. If schools are proactive in addressing mental health, they can serve as crucial intervention points where students learn that it's okay to ask for help, and where they can be directed toward supportive resources, including therapy.

## Mental Health Education and Counseling in Schools

One way schools can initiate mental health conversations in Black households is by embedding mental health education into the curriculum. Classes on emotional intelligence, stress management, conflict resolution, and coping mechanisms for anxiety or depression can help normalize discussions about mental health and give students the language and tools they need to identify when they are struggling. This proactive approach not only prepares students to manage their own mental health but also equips them with knowledge they can take home and share with their families.

Schools that provide access to counselors, social workers, or school psychologists can play an essential role in identifying early signs of mental health struggles in students. In many cases, students may feel more comfortable opening up to a school counselor than to their family members, particularly if therapy and mental health discussions are stigmatized at home. School counselors can serve as a bridge, helping students understand their emotions and directing them to further resources, such as therapy.

For Black youth, culturally competent counseling is crucial. Schools that prioritize hiring counselors who are trained in cultural competence and understand the unique challenges Black students face can create safer and more supportive environments. These counselors can help students address the pressures of living in a racially biased society, cope with discrimination, and navigate their identities. By creating a culture of emotional support within schools, these professionals can also encourage Black students to talk to their parents about mental health, slowly breaking down the stigma surrounding therapy in Black households.

## Involving Families in Mental Health Education

Schools can also take an active role in involving families in mental health advocacy. This could be done through parent workshops, community events, and open forums where mental health professionals educate parents on the importance of mental health care, how to recognize the signs of mental distress in their children, and how to support their child's emotional well-being. For Black families, these events could specifically address cultural barriers to mental health care and provide information on how therapy can help Black youth navigate the challenges of growing up in a racially biased society.

By fostering partnerships between schools and families, educators can help initiate conversations about mental health that extend beyond the classroom. When families see schools prioritizing mental health and promoting therapy as a beneficial resource, they may become more open to discussing these topics at home and more willing to seek therapy when necessary.

# Churches and Community Centers as Safe Spaces for Mental Health

## The Influence of Churches in Black Communities

Churches have long been central to Black communities, serving as not only places of worship but also as social, cultural, and political hubs. Historically, Black churches have been a source of strength and resilience, providing emotional and spiritual support in times of hardship. Given their influence and the trust they have within Black communities, churches are uniquely positioned to become advocates for mental health and therapy.

For many Black individuals, mental health struggles are often addressed through prayer, faith, and spiritual guidance. While faith can be a powerful source of comfort, it's important for Black churches to also acknowledge the need for professional mental health care when necessary. By encouraging members to seek both spiritual and therapeutic support, churches can help destigmatize therapy and create a more holistic approach to mental health.

# Faith-Based Mental Health Initiatives

Many Black churches are already beginning to partner with mental health professionals to provide education and resources to their congregations. Faith-based mental health initiatives can take many forms, including workshops, sermons that address the importance of mental health, or collaborations with local therapists to provide counseling services directly through the church. These initiatives help bridge the gap between faith and therapy, showing that seeking professional help is not a contradiction to faith but a complement to spiritual well-being.

Pastors and faith leaders can play a key role in normalizing mental health discussions by openly addressing mental health issues in their sermons or personal testimonies. When faith leaders speak openly about mental health struggles, it can reduce the shame or embarrassment that many churchgoers may feel about seeking therapy. Pastors can also create opportunities for congregants to ask questions about mental health and provide guidance on how to find culturally competent therapists who align with their spiritual values.

## Creating Safe Spaces in the Church

Churches can create safe spaces for mental health conversations by providing support groups, prayer circles, or small discussion groups focused on mental well-being. These spaces allow members to share their emotional struggles, receive support, and feel heard without fear of judgment. Faith-based support groups that are led by trained mental health professionals or facilitators can help integrate discussions of faith and therapy, making both feel accessible and complementary.

Churches can also provide access to professional counseling services, either by hiring therapists to work directly within the church or by partnering with local mental health organizations. These services can be especially beneficial for congregants who may feel more comfortable seeking therapy through their church community than through outside providers. By offering therapy as part of the church's services, churches help reduce barriers to accessing care, particularly for those who may face financial constraints or mistrust of outside institutions.

## Community Centers as Mental Health Advocates

In addition to churches, community centers are another crucial resource for mental health support in Black neighborhoods. Community centers provide a wide range of services, from after-school programs and job training to health education and social services. By integrating mental health care into their offerings, community centers can help make therapy and emotional support more accessible to Black families.

Community centers can partner with mental health professionals to provide counseling services, workshops, and support groups for individuals of all ages. These programs can focus on topics such as stress management, coping with trauma, navigating racial discrimination, and building emotional resilience. For Black youth in particular, community centers can serve as a safe space to discuss mental health issues and receive support outside of the school or home environment.

## Community Mental Health Advocacy

Community centers can also serve as advocates for mental health by promoting mental health education and awareness. Hosting mental health fairs, wellness events, or community forums can help break down the stigma surrounding therapy and encourage Black families to seek out the support they need. These events can feature mental health professionals, workshops on self-care and emotional health, and information on how to access therapy services in the community.

By collaborating with schools, churches, and mental health professionals, community centers can create a network of support that addresses the emotional needs of Black individuals and families. This holistic approach helps ensure that mental health care is accessible, culturally relevant, and normalized within the community.

# Conclusion

Schools, churches, and community centers have the power to play a transformative role in mental health advocacy for Black families. Schools, as the first point of contact for many children, can help initiate conversations about mental health and therapy, providing education and counseling services that normalize emotional well-being. Churches, long seen as pillars of strength in Black communities, can bridge the gap between faith and therapy by creating safe spaces for mental health discussions and partnering with mental health professionals. Community centers can complement these efforts by offering accessible mental health resources and acting as advocates for emotional health in the community.

By working together, these institutions can break down the stigma surrounding therapy and mental health care, creating a supportive and informed network for Black families. This partnership between schools, churches, and community centers is essential for fostering a culture where mental health is prioritized, therapy is normalized, and Black individuals are empowered to seek the care they deserve.

# Conclusion: Paving the Way for the Next Generation

## From Silence to Conversation

Throughout history, mental health in Black households has often been a topic cloaked in silence. Cultural expectations, mistrust of mental health institutions, and the enduring legacy of trauma have contributed to this silence. For generations, Black individuals and families have been expected to persevere through immense hardships without acknowledging the emotional toll of these experiences. This has led to a harmful cycle of emotional suppression and untreated mental health struggles.

However, as we have explored in this book, breaking the silence around mental health is not only necessary but transformative. By opening up conversations about mental health and embracing therapy as a tool for healing, we have the opportunity to change the narrative for future generations. Speaking openly about mental health can lead to collective healing within families and communities. It allows Black individuals to reclaim their emotional well-being, validate their experiences, and seek the support they deserve.

This shift—from silence to conversation—creates a ripple effect. When one person in a family begins to talk openly about their mental health, it can encourage others to do the same. By normalizing discussions about therapy and mental health, we break down the stigma that has prevented many Black families from accessing the care they need. In this way, vulnerability becomes a form of strength, and emotional openness becomes a pathway to healing.

The importance of this shift cannot be overstated. Mental health affects every aspect of life— relationships, career, physical health, and overall quality of life. When Black families make mental health a priority, they lay the foundation for stronger, healthier, and more resilient communities. By breaking the silence around mental health, we pave the way for future generations to grow up in environments where emotional well-being is valued and supported.

# A Call to Action: Shifting the Culture

The journey toward normalizing mental health care in Black households is not one that can be undertaken by individuals alone. It requires a collective effort from families, communities, and institutions to shift the culture and make therapy an accepted and celebrated part of Black life. This is a call to action for everyone—parents, educators, faith leaders, community organizers, and public figures—to take responsibility for creating a culture that prioritizes emotional well-being and supports mental health care.

## Families: Lead with Vulnerability

The first step begins at home. Families must commit to leading with vulnerability and breaking down the cultural barriers that have stigmatized therapy for so long. This means creating spaces where children and adults alike feel safe expressing their emotions without fear of judgment. Parents and guardians, in particular, have a responsibility to model emotional openness for their children. By sharing their own mental health journeys and encouraging their children to speak openly about their feelings, families can foster an environment where therapy is viewed as a valuable tool for self-care.

## Communities: Build Networks of Support

Communities play a vital role in supporting mental health. Churches, community centers, and local organizations must continue to create safe spaces for mental health discussions and advocate for mental health resources. Community leaders can help reduce the stigma around therapy by promoting mental health education, providing access to culturally competent therapists, and partnering with mental health professionals to offer support services. By building strong networks of support, communities can ensure that mental health care is accessible to all, regardless of socioeconomic status or cultural background.

## Institutions: Advocate for Change

Institutions, including schools, healthcare systems, and the media, have the power to shape public perceptions of mental health. Schools must continue to integrate mental health education into their curricula, providing students with the tools they need to navigate their emotions and seek help when needed. Healthcare systems must prioritize culturally competent care, ensuring that Black individuals receive treatment that is respectful of their experiences and sensitive to their unique challenges. The media must continue to showcase positive representations of mental health and therapy, helping to normalize these conversations in Black households.

## Public Figures: Use Your Platform

Black celebrities, influencers, and public figures have the unique ability to shape culture and influence millions of people. By using their platforms to speak openly about mental health and therapy, they can help normalize these conversations and encourage others to seek support. Public figures who share their own mental health journeys help reduce stigma, showing that therapy is not a sign of weakness but a powerful tool for growth and healing. As more Black public figures embrace therapy, they contribute to shifting the cultural narrative and making mental health a priority in Black communities.

## A New Legacy for the Next Generation

Ultimately, the goal is to create a new legacy for the next generation—one where mental health is not only accepted but celebrated as an essential part of life. By shifting the culture around mental health, we ensure that Black children grow up in environments where they feel supported in expressing their emotions and seeking help when needed. This cultural shift can prevent the emotional suppression and untreated trauma that has affected previous generations, allowing the next generation to thrive emotionally, mentally, and physically.

The work of normalizing mental health care in Black households is ongoing, but it is essential for the well-being of future generations. As we continue to break the silence, build support systems, and embrace therapy, we create a path toward healing for ourselves and for those who come after us. This is the future we must work toward—a future where Black families are empowered to prioritize their mental health, and where therapy is seen as a tool for strength, resilience, and collective healing.

Let us commit to this work. Let us shift the culture, break the silence, and create a new legacy of mental wellness for the Black community.

# Appendix

## Mental Health Resources for Black Families

This comprehensive list includes culturally competent therapists, organizations, and online platforms that specifically support Black mental health. These resources provide access to therapists who understand the unique cultural and social challenges Black individuals face, as well as platforms dedicated to promoting mental wellness in Black communities.

## Culturally Competent Therapy Directories

1. **Therapy for Black Girls**
   A popular online directory that connects Black women with culturally competent therapists. Founded by Dr. Joy Harden Bradford, the platform offers a directory of therapists, as well as resources like podcasts and blog posts about mental health topics relevant to Black women.
   **Website**: therapyforblackgirls.com

2. **Therapy for Black Men**
This platform is dedicated to helping Black men access culturally competent mental health professionals. The directory includes therapists who specialize in issues unique to Black men and provides support to break the stigma surrounding therapy in Black communities.
**Website**: therapyforblackmen.org

3. **National Queer and Trans Therapists of Color Network (NQTTCN)**
A resource for queer and trans people of color, including Black individuals, seeking culturally competent and affirming therapists. NQTTCN focuses on healing within LGBTQ+ communities of color and provides a directory of mental health professionals.
**Website**: nqttcn.com

4. **Inclusive Therapists**
Inclusive Therapists is a directory that focuses on promoting equity, justice, and cultural competence in mental health care. It offers a wide range of therapists who specialize in working with marginalized communities, including Black individuals.
**Website**: inclusivetherapists.com

5. **Open Path Collective**
Open Path connects individuals and families with affordable mental health care by offering a directory of therapists who provide sessions at reduced rates. Many of the listed therapists are culturally competent

and experienced in working with Black clients.
**Website**: openpathcollective.org

6. **Psychology Today Therapist Directory**
A widely used directory that allows users to filter for therapists by race, specialization, and location. Many Black therapists and culturally competent therapists are listed on the platform.
**Website**: psychologytoday.com

7. **BetterHelp**
An online therapy platform that connects individuals with licensed therapists through video, phone, or messaging. While not exclusively for Black clients, BetterHelp offers a diverse pool of therapists and allows users to find culturally competent professionals who meet their needs.
**Website**: betterhelp.com

# Mental Health Organizations for Black Communities

1. **The Boris Lawrence Henson Foundation**
Founded by actress Taraji P. Henson, this foundation is dedicated to eradicating the stigma surrounding mental health issues in the Black community. The organization provides mental health resources, therapy scholarships, and advocacy for culturally competent care.
**Website**: borislhensonfoundation.org

2.  **Black Mental Health Alliance (BMHA)**
    BMHA offers mental health education, advocacy, and support services for Black communities. The organization also provides a referral network for culturally competent therapists.
    **Website**: blackmentalhealth.com

3.  **The Steve Fund**
    This organization focuses on supporting the mental health of young people of color, particularly Black youth. The Steve Fund offers resources, educational programs, and partnerships with colleges and universities to address the mental health needs of students.
    **Website**: stevefund.org

4.  **Black Emotional and Mental Health Collective (BEAM)**
    BEAM is a national training, movement-building, and grant-making organization dedicated to the healing, wellness, and liberation of Black and marginalized communities. The collective provides training, workshops, and resources for both mental health professionals and the public.
    **Website**: beam.community

## Online Platforms and Podcasts

1.  **The Friend Zone Podcast**
    A weekly podcast that discusses mental health, wellness, and pop culture from a Black perspective. Hosts explore a range of topics related to emotional well-being,

relationships, and self-care.
**Website**: loudspeakersnetwork.com/show/
the-friend-zone

2.  **Therapy for Black Girls Podcast**
    Hosted by Dr. Joy Harden Bradford, this
    podcast offers expert insights on mental
    health, personal development, and self-
    care. The episodes are designed to provide
    practical mental health tips while
    normalizing therapy in Black communities.
    **Website**: therapyforblackgirls.com/podcast

3.  **Black Mental Health Matters**
    An online platform and podcast that offers
    discussions on mental health challenges
    within the Black community, featuring
    interviews with mental health professionals,
    advocates, and individuals sharing their
    stories.
    **Website**:
    blackmentalhealthmatters.carrd.co

# Further Reading

## Books on Black Mental Health and Therapy

1. **"The Unapologetic Guide to Black Mental Health" by Dr. Rheeda Walker**
   This book addresses the unique challenges Black people face regarding mental health and provides guidance on how to seek help and thrive emotionally. It also explores the stigma around mental health in Black communities and offers solutions for overcoming it.
2. **"Shook One: Anxiety Playing Tricks on Me" by Charlamagne Tha God**
   In this memoir, Charlamagne Tha God shares his experiences with anxiety and therapy, offering insight into how Black men can overcome the stigma of mental health care and take charge of their emotional well-being.
3. **"Sister Outsider" by Audre Lorde**
   This collection of essays and speeches by Black feminist, poet, and activist Audre Lorde touches on themes of identity, intersectionality, and self-care, providing a profound exploration of how Black women can resist systemic oppression while nurturing their own mental health.

4.  **"My Grandmother's Hands" by Resmaa Menakem**
    A book that explores the trauma Black individuals carry in their bodies due to centuries of systemic racism, "My Grandmother's Hands" provides insight into how trauma manifests physically and emotionally and offers techniques for healing through somatic practices.

## Articles on Black Mental Health

1.  **"The Strong Black Woman Fallacy" by Kendra Cherry (Verywell Mind)**
    This article explores the "strong Black woman" stereotype and its impact on mental health, discussing why Black women often feel pressure to maintain emotional resilience and how therapy can help dismantle these harmful expectations.
2.  **"Black Mental Health Matters: How Racism Impacts Mental Health in the Black Community" (National Alliance on Mental Illness - NAMI)**
    This article highlights the ways systemic racism, generational trauma, and everyday microaggressions affect the mental health of Black people and emphasizes the importance of culturally competent care.

## Documentaries on Black Mental Health

1.  **"The Me You Can't See" (Produced by Oprah Winfrey and Prince Harry)**

This documentary series delves into mental health issues across various communities, including discussions on the impact of systemic racism on Black mental health. Several Black public figures share their personal stories of mental health challenges and therapy.

2.  **"A Conversation About Mental Health in Black America" (PBS)**
    This documentary explores the mental health crisis in Black communities and discusses the cultural and systemic barriers to accessing mental health care. It features interviews with mental health professionals, community leaders, and individuals sharing their experiences with therapy.

By utilizing these resources and engaging with further reading materials, Black families and individuals can access the tools, knowledge, and support they need to prioritize mental health and therapy in their lives. These resources offer a pathway to healing, empowerment, and emotional well-being in Black communities.